EMILY NASH

Just A Few Bumps

First edition

Editing by Hugh Barker
Proofreading by Leslie Kirton

This book was professionally typeset on Reedsy.
Find out more at reedsy.com

This book is dedicated to Mum and Dad. Thank you for supporting me in everything I do.

To Chris, thank you for putting up with the late night calls, the tears, the rants and most of all the endless supply of wine that was needed to write this book.

Contents

I

First Year Student Paramedic

1

What You're About To Read Is Not A Medical Textbook

I started writing this book when I was fresh out of University, filled with the thoughts of where my new and exciting career would take me. What would I see? Who would I help? Will I actually save anyone's life? Writing this book was fun – an escape for me. Little did I know that writing this book would help me through depression, PTSD – and to top it all off – coming back to work, after being signed off for my mental health, I was greeted with a global pandemic. Otherwise known as Covid-19.

I had an idea of what I wanted this book to be – a journal of the emotions I felt throughout my journey to becoming a paramedic and the few years following my qualification. I didn't want to impress people with my academic knowledge or fit in as many big words as I could; I just wanted to describe the highs and low, and the realities of being a paramedic.

Everyone is different and everyone faces different challenges.

I want to talk about the scary jobs, the sad jobs, the happy ones and the downright annoying ones. Every day is different in this line of work and it is a privilege to experience them. If I had realised all those years ago that I was going to actually write this book (and not just toy with the idea of doing it) I would have endless notes and scribbles about all the weird and wonderful things I have seen and done. However, I have my memories – and let's be honest, the weird and wonderful moments are usually the hardest ones to forget.

So, welcome on this trip down memory lane! Of course, to protect the identity of my patients and colleagues, names and ages have been changed. But the patients are real and so are the emotions – both theirs and mine.

THE MOMENT I KNEW

The first time I thought about writing this book was during my first year as a student paramedic. I had just finished a job (a stabbing) in central London, which had nearly taken the life of a young man trying to leave a club. I walked out of the hospital and lit a cigarette, looked down at the blood that was covering my uniform and thought to myself, there and then, in a moment in time that will stay with me: *I should write this down.* This idea was left at that and I continued with my life. When the idea started to really become a reality was after my first shift as a qualified paramedic. My first ever job, my first ever patient. He was dying, choking, lungs full of fluid. I was alone with the patient in the back of the truck (ambulance) and prayed every second he was with me that I could keep him alive that little bit longer. I drove home and thought to myself, *I need my memories to be out on paper, they cannot just be lost to my mind and memory.*

That night I went home and started typing.

NEVER IN MY WILDEST DREAMS

So, as you may have gathered, I am a paramedic. I spent three years training at University, and have been qualified and out on the road for roughly two years. When I was in first year, I remember being completely in the dark about what my placements would entail and what would be expected of me. I searched the internet for tales and stories from other students as to what it was like, to no avail.

To say I was a novice would be an understatement. I didn't come from a medical background and, quite frankly, I would never in my wildest dreams have thought that this was to be my future career when I was younger.

Five years on and I am still a novice! There are still many times when I think I don't know what I am doing, and I question myself regularly as to why I dived head-first into such a stressful job. Sometimes I bloody hate my job, but I bloody love it all the same; I want to share the reasons why.

Many people watch *999: What's Your Emergency?* and the hit show *Ambulance.* Don't get me wrong - they're both entertaining to watch. However, there are many aspects to the job that don't get shown in these programs. Having watched shows like this, the first question anyone will ask when they find out I am a paramedic will be: 'What is the worst thing you have seen?'

Every time I am asked this, I take a few seconds to answer, because really, what do they want to hear? Is it the bloody trauma? The mangled bodies? The elderly lady dying alone with no family? A dying child? I mean, it is not going to be the greatest icebreaker no matter what answer I give, but what do people really want to hear?

This is a question that I still don't know how to answer. So instead of trying, why don't I talk firstly about something I *do* know, which is how I got into a paramedic degree with no medical background at all, while watching TV with a cuppa in my hand.

999: WHAT'S YOUR EMERGENCY?

A little about myself first to put this all into context: I was in my early 20s, living in a one-bedroom flat on my own. After a couple of messy breakups I had decided to go it alone with my own place, so I would have my freedom.

I loved living on my own, I have always been happy in my own company and having a place to shut out the world was amazing. I could cook whenever I wanted, stay up as late as I wanted, and clean whenever I wanted. However, to pay for this lovely one bed flat, I needed to work. . . A LOT.

Whenever I wasn't home, I was working. I needed two jobs just to make ends meet. Sadly, this doesn't make me any different from many people who are working on a minimum wage: it is simply not enough to pay your way with one job in this day and age. So, I would work during the day in a mind-numbing office job, where I was underappreciated and seriously underpaid, then three evenings a week and all weekend I would work at a restaurant.

The perks of working at a restaurant, especially at the weekends, were the tips! Often these would double my weekend wages, so I felt I could never give up the restaurant work. Even after spending all that time working, I would still struggle every month to pay all the bills, get the food in and somehow try to fit in a life as well.

Now the thought of a career change often crossed my mind. However, with just a few OK 'A' levels and limited career experience, my chances of bagging myself a new job with a vast pay increase were small. Besides, where would I start?

I had no idea what I wanted to do with myself. All I did know was that I wanted to be proud of the career I made for myself, and I was willing to put in all the effort I could muster to get myself there.

I am sitting on the sofa, cup of tea in hand. It was an evening off work so that involved being in my pyjamas by roughly seven o'clock and bingeing on telly - usually Netflix or streaming something online; but on this night I decided to see what was on Freeview instead.

I'm skipping through the channels and I'm drawn into a programme I've never seen before – *999: What's Your Emergency?* This particular episode follows ambulances on a busy Saturday night. I see the hassle of dealing with one particularly drunk patient, who can barely walk, but he was refusing the help of the ambulance staff.

Knowing what I do now about a busy Saturday night, I know this would have been infuriating the crew working on this job. However, on screen they were calm and patient, walking alongside the guy and trying to inform him of the dangers of walking home alone drunk, (which is a very fair point). If I'm honest I can't really remember how it ended, and whether the drunk guy got in the ambulance or not. But I know the rest of the show focused on the highs and lows of Saturday night drunken punters.

I remember thinking at the time: *that looks quite fun. . . I could do that job, I mean I have a lot of patience and don't mind drunks, so heck... I'll look into it.*

I am not sure why it escaped me that a paramedic's job wouldn't solely consist of picking up drunks off the floor, and that it would be a serious medical profession. But to be frank, I am glad I didn't think it through properly because if I had I wouldn't be a qualified paramedic working for, in my opinion, one of the best ambulance services in the world - The London Ambulance Service.

So, on the morning after my evening of TV bingeing, with a cup of tea back in my hand, I found myself Googling away for courses and instructions on how to become a paramedic. I managed to find a degree course at a local University. I never had been interested in University when I was at school, so when it had been time to look at UCAS points and how to apply I had often just skipped that lesson to go and smoke under the D Block stairs. I know: classy lady! So, when I was looking for this course, I was pretty much in the dark about how the process worked. To make life easier, I decided to just ring the number that was printed below the course description and see what they had to say regarding start dates and qualifying criteria.

This is how the conversation went.

'Hello, Blah Blah Blah University. . . how can I help?'

'Hi there, my name's Emily, I was just looking at your course here for Paramedic Science and was wondering what grades I needed and what the process is for enrolling into something like that?'

'Ahh I see, no problem, just quickly... what grades did you get in GSCE science?'

'Ermmm I did double science and got two C's... I know that's probably not ideal...'

'No that's fine, and A-levels?'

'I got a C in media studies, a B in Art, and C in psychology.'

'That's great. OK, well I can see here that those grades would be enough to get in through clearing if you would like to go ahead?'

Now I was thinking: *1. What on earth is clearing?* and *2. How on earth are those crappy grades good enough for a medical degree?* But still I proceeded.

'Erm, yeah great... sorry... what's clearing?'

'So, clearing is when the deadline for admission is gone for this year's course, however we still have some places available, and people that didn't quite have the grades first time round can apply through clearing. We are actually holding interviews over the phone for clearing now, I can do one with you now if you would like? To see if you would be accepted for a face-to-face interview?'

Well – this has all developed quickly, I thought. *But yeah, why the hell not?*

'Yes please!'

That is how it all began. I had a brief interview over the phone asking me about my character and work ethic and why I was interested in a course like that. Of course, I didn't mention the fact that my whole interest had stemmed from an evening watching TV. Instead, I probably made up some lifelong dream of mine. However, I can easily say that helping people was my career choice. I had always also known I wanted a job that was mentally fulfilling so that, after my hard day's work, I would feel I had made a difference in some way.

Looking back now, maybe this really was the job I was always meant to do. It just took a TV programme to make me see it.

Back to the telephone interview. I must have answered the questions reasonably well, because at the end of the phone call, I was told the interviews would be held a week later at 9am.

At this point it hadn't occurred to any of my friends or family that I was looking at doing a degree and making a complete career change, so to suddenly declare 'right, I'm off for an interview at this University to get myself a career change,' was going to be quite a shock! And to be honest, it was! My friends gave me confused support, saying things like: 'Ahhh… paramedic science… OK where did that come from? Bet you're great, best of luck!'

My parents, on the other hand, looked at me like I was a crazy woman. 'But you can't financially afford to go to University full-time – you have your flat and your jobs. Are you planning on quitting your jobs for this?' These were all questions I hadn't really thought about myself just yet. I was just running with it to see where it went. There was no point stressing about the 'What if's': if I didn't get a place at University then life would just continue as normal.

I vividly remember sitting at a pub having lunch with my Mum after my interviews were done and feeling really anxious about what the final result would be. I really wanted this now. After seeing the lecture rooms and the resus (short for resuscitation) dummies in the skills lab, I was feeling a drive that took me quite by surprise. I was excited.

The look on my Mum's face was priceless. 'Well, this has all happened very quickly… do you really think you can do this?' My mother is the most supportive woman I have ever met: she would have given me the world if I needed it, but she was also a sensible woman and, most of all, a worrier! She worried about everything, and overthought everything.

In her head I was about to quit my jobs, get into debt, find it too difficult (because let's be honest, I had never been an academic in school), quit Uni after a few months and be back to shitty square one. Which was not the craziest of thought patterns. I mean it must have crossed my mind as well at some point, but all I can remember thinking is: *I'll prove you all wrong and I will do this!*

I finally had a real drive and passion for something! I had an overall goal. There was a light at the end of the tunnel... and this was all before I had even stepped into an ambulance.

So, needless to say, I got offered a place at University and I informed my nine-to-five employer with a beaming smile on my face that I would be leaving to attend University in the coming September. Which, much to the annoyance of my employers, was only a month and a half away.

Personally, I was shit-scared. In not much more than a month, I would be attending full-time lectures on medical science and, at some point, I would be given the responsibility of sitting and working in an ambulance in London. But I reassured myself it was all going to be fine – my first placement with LAS (London Ambulance Service) wouldn't be until the following December and I would know at least the basics by then... or enough to get me through the ten weeks... right?

Well, let me tell you, in my first ten weeks on the road as a first-year student I saw some of the sickest patients I've ever seen to this day: some of the most chaotic and disgusting scenes, and downright disturbing ones.

No lecture was going to prepare me for this and I was never going to be ready for it... you just have to go along for the ride.

GOING ALONG FOR THE RIDE

The night before my first shift, I remember sitting in my flat with the guy I was dating at the time and trying to confide in him about how nervous I was. He, unfortunately, was more focused on playing FIFA... but, hey, that gives you an insight as to why we aren't still dating.

I kept overthinking every scenario in my head, like what if they ask me a question and I don't know the answer? Or I can't remember how to do something I am supposed to have been taught? Well, looking back now I wish I could tell myself to bloody relax: *You're a first-year student on your first placement, on your first day! You're not meant to know everything.*

I had already done my practice run for the drive to work, so I knew my way and knew the timings, so I wasn't late. So, all I had to do was wake up on time, and on time I was. In fact, if I recall correctly, I rocked up a nice hour early, just for good measure. Walking into the station for the first time, I kept my head low and made my way to what looked like the kitchen to make myself a cup of coffee and find a safe place to have a cigarette to calm my nerves. As I walked through, I got the friendly smiles and nods from people walking by, which I now know is common courtesy among paramedics or anyone in green – everyone will say hello to everyone. Regardless whether or not you have met this person in green before, you will always smile, wave or say hello.

After glugging my coffee and probably chain-smoking three cigarettes, I bucked up and summoned up the courage to find my mentor for the ten weeks, to begin learning the ropes.

There is a very distinctive sound that an ambulance makes when a job comes in, and when this sound becomes familiar (which doesn't take long) it sends a nervous jolt through your body where, for a split second from when the sound begins and the job appears on the screen, you pause to see what the public has in store for you today.

So, I had found my crew, the truck was ready and the alarm buzzed: it was *'go'* time – the first job came in.

2

Let Your Mind Run Wild

Please feel free to let your mind run wild on this one, because at the time mine was! We had been called to a RTC (road traffic collision). I had visions of people trapped in cars, a bus flipped on its side, and cars all over the road. While all these thoughts were going through my head, my mentor was running through what was needed of me, step by step. I had the sirens buzzing in my ear, and traffic dodging our path which, by the way is bloody amazing to watch from inside the vehicle that has the lights and sirens. All while my mentor was asking me questions like: 'OK what's the first thing you do when arriving on scene?'

'Erm…' There was a blank expression on my face… 'Check for danger?'

'Yes.' This was followed by a slight but friendly laugh. To elaborate, when approaching any job, the first thing any medical professional should check for is: DRABC. D – DANGER. R – RESPONSE. A – AIRWAY. B – BREATHING. C – CIRCULATION. This had been drilled into us on our first few weeks of training and it's pretty much all I could bring to the table right now, apart from maybe CPR (which I had only practised on a dummy).

In training we are taught to vocalise this loudly so our colleagues and trainers can hear. In reality, if I entered a scene now shouting: 'I'm checking for danger!' 'It is all clear, safe to approach!' I would be seen as a complete dick and I would lose all respect in about 20 seconds. This approach is all meant to be done in the quiet of your mind... so that is what I did.

I approached calmly and pragmatically; I assessed the situation and dealt with each patient accordingly... *Cough* did I heck... Actually, we arrived on the scene and I followed my mentor like a lost puppy waiting to be told what to do, because all my training had gone from my mind and I was now just another bystander staring at a car crash by the side of the road.

Thankfully it was not too traumatic; a young mother and father had taken their two-year-old to London Zoo that day and, while driving home, had swerved onto the other side of the road and collided head-on with a double-decker bus.

Now, due to London's 20mph zone and generally dense traffic, the impact had been relatively slow, so apart from just a few bumps and sore necks, everyone was fine. We got the young family, who were at this point standing outside the car, onto the ambulance for a quick check over. Mum was holding onto her son for dear life while he cried. I mean, getting into a car accident is enough to scare any adult, but for a two-year-old it must have been terrifying. He didn't appear to have any injuries but I remember my mentor being very thorough with her examination.

After a chat, and a check on everyone's main vital signs, everything was looking good. However, something was off with the Dad – he appeared like a broken man. It's a harsh description I know, but I remember looking at him and thinking: *You're not telling the truth about this accident.* The police were en route to the crash to take statements and I think this was playing on his mind. So, the initial story told to us was that he wasn't sure how he had drifted onto the other side of the road, it was all 'a bit fuzzy'. He said he thought he had been trying to settle his son in the backseat.

Now, looking at this medically, it was important for us to try to find out why he had a memory block. It could have been for several reasons, including the worst-case scenario of having sustained a head injury. He might have blacked out while driving, causing him to swerve. Then the question would be: 'Why did he black out? Or did it all simply happen a bit too quickly and now his memory is playing tricks about what happened?' It would be in the patient's best interest for the crew to investigate this further, and, as I will elaborate throughout this book, history-taking is the key to any diagnosis. It will create a detailed back story that, nine times out of ten, will bring you to the most likely conclusion about what's going on with a patient.

So, with this guy, let the digging begin...my mentor started...

'Run me through what happened today that led up to the accident, what can you remember?'

'Erm, well... it's my son's birthday so we took him to the zoo... we didn't get much sleep last night because he wasn't really settling, but that's about it.'

'So, you've been there all day... has it been a long drive for you guys?'

'Not overly... we live, like, 30 minutes away.'

'OK, how's your sleep been lately then, you said you didn't get much sleep?'

Now the father starts to cry, only slightly but I see the tears building, and now I know what my mentor is trying to get at.

'Everything you say to us is completely confidential and we don't pass these things onto the police, but it is important for us to have an understanding of why you lost control of the car. There are no judgements here… but Sir, do you think you fell asleep at the wheel?'

His head was down, he didn't make eye contact with her and just nodded. His wife grabbed his hand, almost to say: 'I forgive you, it's OK'. Then the police arrived and, still to this day, I don't know what story he told them, but we had our answers and medically everyone was fine.

I didn't get involved at all with this job but I remember sitting in the corner of the ambulance just listening with so many thoughts rattling through my head: *Is it OK that I feel sorry for this man? How am I going to have this conversation with someone one day? How badly could this have gone? Would I forgive my husband if my child was in the car? … not sure…*

But what I did know was that this job was going to open up everyone's world to me. Up until that point I had known my world and the details of it, but now, every time that alarm buzzed in the ambulance I would be walking into someone else's world, and potentially on the worst day of their lives, with that person expecting you to make it all better again.

BIG SICK

There is a term that is used in medical practice: 'big sick'. It's not the most professional term, granted, however it is how we clinicians describe a patient that needs medical attention immediately. I learnt this term pretty early on in my degree. As a paramedic who practices in emergency medicine, you would think that every patient would be 'big sick.' However, this just isn't the case. I would say a good 80 percent of patients we see don't necessarily need an ambulance, meaning they could have made their own way to the hospital or to their GP because they simply do not need the treatment we provide. Putting it in basic terminology, we get people breathing again, or restart a broken heart, or fix the heart before it breaks. We help with horrendous pain. We stop you bleeding out. We pull out that Brussels sprout or piece of Lego from your airway. You get my gist?

We cannot fix a cough you have had for five days and the antibiotics aren't helping. We can't fix chronic back pain, even though you're still able to function on a day-to-day basis. Of course, there is always going to be the worst-case scenarios, where that stomach ache is a ruptured bowel or that headache is actually a bleed on the brain, which is why we still go to these jobs. But more often, they're not the worst-case scenario. So, when crews do arrive on scene to a 'big sick' patient it's safe to say that most clinicians working the front line will very briefly think… 'Ah, shit,' because we have become conditioned into thinking it's not going to be that bad!

In my first year as a student paramedic, I saw some of the sickest patients I've ever had. Now, is that because I was new to it all and everyone seemed sick? Possibly, but these people will always stick in my mind as the worst; I saw cases of overdose, stabbing, anaphylaxis, P.E (pulmonary embolism), exacerbation of COPD (chronic obstructive pulmonary disease), and domestic abuse cases along with child neglect cases all in my first year. I actually had two bad overdoses in my first year, plus one which we found out afterwards had been an overdose.

18

The first overdose I had ever seen was on my second day when we were called to an elderly gentleman 'acting strange'. A neighbour and friend had called it in.

3

Acting Strange You say?

Now, an elderly man (who happened to be a known alcoholic) acting strangely could have a multiple of causes: he could just be drunk; he could have obtained a urinary tract infection, something which is known to cause a state of delirium; he could have other medical conditions that are affecting his state of mind, such as dementia. So, with this patient, an open mind and a thorough investigation was going to be needed to figure out why he was acting strangely.

Walking into this patient's house was an experience beyond description but I will do my best... The instant odour of faeces and urine was strong and almost unbearable: anyone who didn't need to be in there would have left immediately. It was the kind of smell that would hit your nostrils and get ingrained in your hair. That smell would linger in your clothes and your pores for the rest of the day. The hallway was almost impassable, as we had to clamber across obstacles to get to the stairs. The patient was confined to his bedroom. The bedroom was filled with empty bottles, fag butts, ashtrays, rubbish and filth. The bed that this poor man was lying on was covered in urine and his own faeces and, by the looks of it, none was fresh. He had been living like this for some time. The man himself was dirty and ungroomed. His white beard had turned a shade of brown/yellow. His skin was a mixture of purple and white. There was a pool of black sticky vomit trailing from his mouth to the bed. His eyes were fixed to the ceiling, and he hadn't reacted when we had entered the room. He had a dirty white vest top on and nothing else.

When I think that the friend had only called this in as the patient acting strange, words escape me. The patient was quite clearly 'big sick'. But it still wasn't clear what he had taken that had caused this, or if he had in fact taken anything at all. The evidence for the diagnosis came from the empty packets of drugs lying around the bed, the crack pipe, and alcohol bottles. To this day I don't know what happened. I stood at the bottom of the bed, transfixed by the sight of my mentor and her crewmate trying to get this gentleman off the bed and onto a carry chair so he could be extracted from the house to the truck (ambulance).

The relevant medical interventions were carried out, as I remember them struggling to get a cannula in and to clear his airway to get the oxygen mask on. All the time this was happening I stayed in my position like a spare part, not knowing what the hell I could do to help. I hated it, the feeling of being so useless and, quite frankly, just in the way.

I decided to do the only thing I knew I could do, and that was to clear a path on the stairs and hallway so that once the patient was finally ready to be taken to the truck it could be done a little easier. The patient started to become more vocal once the crew were repositioning him, and he was receiving some oxygen. However, the sounds weren't really like language or anything that could be understood: all I can describe it as is howling. He was groaning and screaming out but the screams were not of fear or pain. They were of anger and confusion. His eyes would fix onto you in a way that made it look like they were piercing right through you. It was terrifying. I remember at the time thinking: *this is what possession looks like*.

That's how he was looking and acting: like he was possessed. That's where the first doubts started setting into my mind, I nearly walked out of the property twice because of the smell, and then on the truck I sat in the furthest seat away. I watched in awe, disturbed, as my mentor tried to suction out the black vomit. Then, on realising that the substance was too thick for the suction machine, she made the brave decision to stick her fingers in this patient's mouth to claw out the thick, foul-smelling substance.

I really questioned whether I could ever do that. It's safe to say that now I know I can, and I have dealt with similar situations. However, I believed at the time it was more the uselessness that I struggled with. I was watching a man die and there was nothing I could do about it. We took him in blued (which means taking someone to hospital with the blue lights on) and handed over to the resus team waiting for us at the hospital. Afterwards we went back to our truck, cleaned up the remnants of the chaotic scene and carried on with our day, never finding out whether this man lived to see another day.

Now I apologise if these first few jobs I am describing are lacking the medical evidence they deserve. However, at the time I had a very basic understanding of what was going on.

When numbers appeared on the screen that would theoretically tell me the patients' observations like heart rate, blood pressure, or oxygen levels I would generally go off my mentor's facial expression to see if it was a good or bad result.

I think it is good to be made aware that most students like to act like they know what they are doing, even though they probably don't and are learning every single day. Even now, as a fully qualified paramedic I am still learning every single day. I will see something new on the road that baffles me, and then I will have to go and research it after the job is done. If you come across something you've never seen before on the road, the best way I can put it is you simply have to roll with the punches.

Speaking of rolling with the punches, next I will describe a situation where I found myself seriously out of my depth, in a situation that was, quite frankly, dangerous. This was my first stabbing.

4

Welcome To The Big City

A night shift can go many ways, especially on a weekend. Sometimes you see nothing but drunken punters who have had a little too much that evening, and now their friends think they are unconscious and dying, or else they have had a fall and lost a sizeable chunk of a body part. Fights are also a common one: on average you will see significantly more trauma on a weekend night shift. But this didn't seem to be the case during this particular night shift.

At the beginning, it was just a normal run of the mill shift: until it reached about 3:30am, when we had a job come down on the vehicle's computer. We were being sent to a stabbing of a 30-year-old male. Police were on the scene and requesting immediate back-up from the ambulance service. The adrenaline had started to run through my body as this was my first ever stabbing and I had no idea what to expect. I was a week into my training and my mentor had started training me on how to attend a job. This essentially means you're running the job: you greet the patient first, hear the story, and come up with a treatment plan.

You write the paperwork and hand over the patient at hospital. The other crewmate at this time will get obs (observations) for you, get the necessary kit that you need and basically be there to assist you. (Well, that's the general idea but most teams will all pitch in anywhere we can). Usually on a shift, one member will attend the first half of the shift and the other will drive, and then they will swap over. As I was a student and still learning I would be attending all shift. Also, I couldn't drive so there wasn't much else for me to do. So, this job was 'mine' – I say this lightly as my mentor was always shadowing everything I did, since I am working under their registration, which pretty much means that what they say goes.

There are certain jobs that make the driver really kick in their blue light driving and this was definitely one of them. As we steamed through the city trying to get to the job the vehicle radio went to open mic. Usually when someone wants to speak to control, they ring up on a closed channel, so you're talking privately with the person sat in the control room. However, this was being broadcast to everyone on that channel. Whether this was done in a panic or to save time, I do not know.

'X111, I am going to need HEMS on this job immediately.'

OK, so let's break this down: X111 is the call sign that all crews or single responders will use: they will all have a different call sign for that shift and that is what we refer to ourselves as. 'HEMS' are known as the grown-ups of trauma: they usually consist of an A&E doctor and advanced paramedic who work in a separate car or helicopter and come out for difficult trauma jobs.

This told us straight away it was going to be a bad one. Now of course we didn't know this was for our job, but we had a pretty good guess that it was. On arrival we found the area swarming with police. And when I say police, I mean police fully kitted out with riot shields. There must have been four to five cars, three or four police vans, and two riot vans – giant blue and grey police riot vans that look pretty intimidating.

The scene looked insane. My crewmates put on their stab-proof vests. Of course, as a student I didn't have one so I went without. We jumped out of the truck and my crewmates grabbed the necessary kit. While they were doing this, an extremely flushed police officer came up to me and shouted: 'Who is attending this?' Well stupid old me raised my hand in response to his question without really thinking it through.

'Right guys bubble her and take her in.'

'Excuse me bubble what?' Next thing I knew I had been surrounded by police with riot shields and was being pushed through a crowd of extremely drunk and angry partygoers. Hands were reaching over the police shields and I wasn't sure if they were trying to hit me, grab me or what was going on. I got nearer to the patient and a police officer that was next to the patient, also surrounded by what looked like 50 people screaming and shouting, made eye contact with me. He reached out, grabbed my arm and pulled me through the crowd, pushing people left right and centre. The paramedic on the car treating this patient must have been so relieved to see someone else in green, and then so fucked off to see a student standing there holding a bottle of Entonox and nothing else: Entonox was bringing absolutely nothing to the table here. It is essentially laughing gas which women have when giving birth. It is an effective pain relief for mild to moderate pain. I searched frantically for my mentor and her crewmate but they were nowhere to be seen, so it was time to put on my big boy pants and get stuck in.

'How can I help?' This male, who was probably in his 30s, was sitting by a shop door outside a nightclub with a 6-inch laceration down and across his throat. There was blood all over his shirt and body. Family members and an extremely distraught young lady were screaming in our faces telling us we need to help him.

'Get something to stop the bleeding out and I'll sort the oxygen out' shouted the paramedic over the screams.

'OK.' I started to rip open the bags in a blind panic trying to see what might be best to cover this large wound and stop the bleeding, all while being as quick as I can. I found a Russell bandage and ripped it open, hoping this would do the trick. I leaned over the patient and slammed it to his neck while the paramedic fitted some oxygen through a high-flow face mask. That's a key aspect to any big trauma job: stop the bleeding, apply oxygen at 15L, get a line in through a cannula in case fluids or other medication and RUN. By this time, my mentor and crewmate had managed to battle their way through the crowd and had a carry chair in hand. I managed to get the man's name... but for now we will call him John.

'John, we need to get you on the chair and get you to the ambulance, can you stand?'

'Just leave me to die, I want to die!'

'John, you don't want to die and you're not going to, so get up and let's go'

'Leave me, I'M DYING, I'M DYING!'

A screaming, intoxicated woman stepped in: 'Why are you not helping him... HELP HIM, OMG stop it... they're letting him die!'

Police: 'Everyone get back now, GET BACK.' Some pushing and shoving started and it was getting way too hairy for me and everyone else in green, it's time to get the hell out of this!

'Everyone, lift him now! We're going,' John got dragged onto the chair and the police formed another bubble of shields around us and ran us back to the truck. HEMS were waiting by the truck, ready to receive a handover and help out where they could. We managed to get John onto the bed. He was now a fraction calmer and asking us to save him and not let him die, which was an improvement. I was told to cut off all his clothing to see if there were more stab wounds. Stab victims often don't feel the second or third knife wound, because their sole attention is on the first. I started cutting off his shirt by slicing straight up the middle. The torso seemed to be clear but there was so much blood on the torso, we all thought there must be more stab wounds. I sliced the sleeves to the shirt and revealed five stab wounds down the right arm and one to the right side of his rib cage.

The one to the rib cage was a serious concern, he could have punctured a lung and that would affect his oxygen levels and his ability to breathe. He was still on the high flow of oxygen and his oxygen levels were staying at a stable rate. To everyone's amazement, his blood pressure was OK: not great but manageable. He had bilateral cannulas placed in both arms with fluid running through them. All the bleeding had stopped and everything was bandaged up. The rise and fall of his chest we watched closely but there was no deterioration.

With HEMS on board, two flushed paramedics, one emergency technician, one screaming patient, police sitting in front and an escort traveling behind – and lastly a very flustered me, we headed off to one of the major London trauma centres on blue lights. I was talking to John throughout the journey, reassuring him, attempting to calm him and talking about his little boy, who was going to be three years old soon. I attempted to ask him what happened that led to this horrific attack and this was his answer:

'I was walking out of the bar and this guy was hitting on my cousin. Her boyfriend started to kick off with the guy so I went in between them to calm the situation and the next thing I knew someone got me from behind and sliced a knife along my throat. Then I felt a burning sensation down my arm and thought they had thrown acid or something down me but I couldn't see anything. Next thing I knew I was on the floor with you guys. Like what the fuck... I was trying to stop the fight and I got fucked up for it.'

He went on to start crying, wiping his eyes hard: he kept repeating that he wasn't a fighter and this shouldn't have happened. Which I completely agreed with.

We got him into the trauma centre and the HEMS doctor handed over to the trauma team waiting in resus. We said our goodbyes and best wishes and departed back to the truck to catch our breath and gather our thoughts.

We sat there for a good 30 minutes chatting about what had just happened and cleaning the blood off ourselves and the equipment. By this point I just needed a cigarette and some time alone. I walked out of the truck and along the building to the smoking area.

Then, ahead of me I heard this panicked mumbling noise. I looked closer and saw two women in their glittery dresses and platform heels attempting to hold up a man.

What on earth?

'Help us please!' The two women came up to me and were in clear view. The young male was slumped, with one arm over each of the lady's shoulders and blood down his face.

29

'Please... he has been stabbed!'

'Oh, for fuck's sake!' Not professional, granted, but professionalism had gone for me at this point. I tilted the guy's head back to check his response and there was a fresh puncture wound under his left eye where he had been stabbed in the face. His left eye was bulging and bloodshot. I grabbed the male from the girls' arms and rushed him inside, told the girls to wait where they were, then took him into resus hanging off my shoulder.

'Erm... help please... this guy's been stabbed.'

'This guy just came up to me outside the front doors!'

Nurses and doctors looked on in surprise and disbelief, then quickly reacted to take the male off my hands and strip him down to assess further. I waited with him briefly, feeling I had some sort of duty to this guy.

He thankfully had no other injuries and apart from potentially losing his eye (which had yet to be established) he was stable. Unfortunately, he wasn't my patient so we had to leave to continue our shift. I walked out back to my truck and told the team debriefing in the truck what had just happened.

'Well, a night like this doesn't happen often,' they said – God, how I wish that statement was still the truth, but times are changing.

Welcome to London on a Saturday night.

After that job, I reflected on my approach. I had so badly wanted to be a part of the action, which seemed like something out of a TV crime drama, but in fact I had put myself in danger and put my mentor at risk, since I was her responsibility. Luckily, I hadn't ended up getting hurt and the patient had survived. However, I had to remind myself that night that I wasn't a medic and I was there to learn.

However, I did leave that shift with a buzz, almost like the adrenaline was still coursing through my veins at the prospect that this was going to be my actual job.

How exciting it all was, I thought at the time. Oh, how I wished I had someone waiting for me at home so I could tell them all about it.

5

So, What's Actually The Problem Here?

Now it is true that your sickest patients always stick with you, embedded in your memory. However, some of the less sick patients also tend to stick in your memory, for very different reasons. There are some call outs we go to as ambulance staff that leave us scratching our heads and wondering: *Why on earth was an emergency ambulance just called to this person?*

For example, there was a point when I realised that not every patient is going to be unwell. Some people just like to know that we will arrive regardless. This happened when we were called to a woman in her 50s who had just got home from her GP's surgery and was complaining of high blood pressure. We arrived on scene to find a woman sitting in her arm chair smoking a cigarette.

'Hello Mary, what seems to be the problem today?'

'I need you to do my blood pressure'

'OK. Do you suffer from high blood pressure?'

'I DONT KNOW!'

'What do you mean, why do you think your blood pressure is high?'

'I don't but the doctor wouldn't check it when I went to see him today.'

'Wait… let me get this correct, so you called an ambulance because the doctor wouldn't do your blood pressure, also you are not diagnosed with high blood pressure?'

'Yes.'

'Mary, this is not something to call an emergency ambulance out for… we will have to do other checks on you also if you want an assessment.'

'No, nothing else needs to be checked. I'm fine. Just do my blood pressure and then leave, please.'

Well, at least she was being polite about it. I got my manual blood pressure gauge out because, to be honest, the practice was good for me.

'It's all good, Mary.'

'Thank you, you can go now.' I looked at my mentor, wondering: *Do we just leave?*

'OK, I need you to sign the back of our paperwork, and state you have declined the rest of our checks. Is that OK, Mary?'

'Yes, that's fine dear, thank you. Bye.' By this point I was completely confused. I felt as if this woman needed a strongly worded conversation about wasting the emergency services' time. However, some battles just aren't worth fighting and after a quick bit of paperwork we were ready to go off again to another job.

6

The Tye Dye Effect

There are many parts to this job: it's not all medical. There's a massive social factor to this job that no one ever really trains for. You either have the ability to talk to people or you have to learn fast. You need to be able to talk on a level that the individual understands – the conversation is often sensitive and needs a certain level of grace, patience, understanding, empathy and confidence in what you are saying. This is an attribute I felt I had well before the medical knowledge, I have always had the ability to empathise with people; you might say I am a 'people person'.

I think during the first year of training that is something I could provide with confidence. The true challenge is trying to connect and show an understanding of how a person is feeling – when you have never personally been in the same situation.

One time, we got called to help a 29-year-old woman after an assault. She was in her home and police were already on the scene. She was accompanied by her very friendly and smiley three-year-old son. When we got to the metal gate at the front entrance to her house, a policeman was standing on the inside of the gate. So, you would assume the metal gate was open... but you would be wrong. The gate was locked and no one had the key to open it. The boyfriend of the patient had beaten her black and blue and then locked her in the property with her son. The police had managed to climb this metal gate and fit through the gap at the top, so we followed suit.

They were in the process of getting the gate unlocked, but if the police could climb over it then so could we. We entered the property and found the patient chatting to police; she was clearly shaken up but, considering the circumstances, seemed to be coping quite well. Maybe this wasn't the first time – statistically it probably wasn't. Domestic assaults are rarely one-off incidents and are usually part of a pattern of abusive and controlling behaviour.

This was a nice home. You could see this woman clearly took pride in her home and the happiness of her child. There were toys, drawings, and photos on display to brighten things up. Among the picture-perfect ideology of this home was the trail of a brutal and savage fight. Furniture was overturned, chairs lying askew, and some kind of substance (at this point unidentified) was all across the floor. However, from the nose-burning stench of bleach, I could have a pretty good guess as to what the substance was on the floor.

On getting closer to the patient, I could see the physical damage this man had done. She had cuts all down her arms, chucks of hair missing, and jagged lacerations to her throat. Her hair was clumped together and starting to turn green in patches. Her clothes had taken on a tie-dye effect where the bleach was changing the colour of the fabric. Before I had a chance to introduce myself to the patient her son came up to me to show us his new truck toy and ask us to come and play.

'Oh wow, that looks cool. Not right now… shall we see Mummy first?' He smiled and sweetly walked off back to the police officer who had been giving him his undivided attention. I approached to interrupt the conversation between the patient and the police officer taking his report.

'Sorry to interrupt guys, hi there, I'm sorry we are here today, how can we help, I can see some cuts… are there any other injuries?'

'Hi. Thanks for coming guys, I'm OK really… they're not that deep. I'd quite like to wash the bleach out of my hair.'

'Yes of course, how does your skin feel? Is there any burning?'

'No, it just feels irritated, if I'm honest,' she held back her emotions and wiped her arms down.

The police officer said she could run her hair under the sink if she wanted.

'Yes, sorry. I just want to make sure you've not got any bleach in your mouth or eyes, and that your skin's not burning.'

'I'm honestly OK, I know you guys need to come and make sure I'm all right. I just want to get out of here as he might come back.'

'Ma'am if he comes back, we are here and he will be arrested immediately,' said the policeman, 'but if I'm honest he will see the police cars and I can't imagine he will come here. We have officers trying to find him now.'

'That worries me more. What if you don't find him and he knows I have called you. This is just going to make things worse.'

My protective instincts kicked in – all I wanted to say is: 'That man won't get to you, you are safe now and you have completely done the right thing by calling the police.' But if

I'm honest, in my naivety, I didn't know how this worked and whether she really was going to be safe now. The worst thing I could have done is to start spouting some promise that I myself had no control over.

'Can you run over everything that happened today, I'm sorry you have to go over it all again, but I need a proper picture of what has happened so we can assess you properly.'

'OK, shall we sit?' We all sit calmly, but with a dark cloud looming because we all know this is going to be hard to hear. She begins by telling us how the argument came about and how it all seemed to be run of the mill couple bickering. However, it had taken a turn when the partner had started accusing her of being unfaithful. I can't recall the reasons behind his thought process but I do remember thinking they were completely bizarre. He had tried to grab her phone, which she resisted – he had reacted to this act of defiance by punching her round the face, which had probably caused the black eye she was developing. He had then continued to grab her by the hand and drag her around the living area a few times while shouting abuse at her.

The son, who was also in the living room, had bravely shouted at his Dad and tried to get him to stop pulling Mommy's hair. Dad then decided to push his son so hard that he flew over the dining room chair which was placed on the far side of the room, and was now on its side in the corner.

This was our patient's breaking point and she had tried to fight back. Kicking and screaming she had tried to break out of his grasp. At this point he had grabbed a knife, pinned her to the ground and slowly sliced the knife back and forth over her neck. Not enough to draw serious blood but enough to cut. It was a sick and twisted game he had been playing to scare this woman to death without reaching that actual outcome.

From the lacerations to her hands and arms the patient had clearly tried to fight herself free. Then she had lain, bloody and terrified, while her partner went and grabbed a bottle of bleach from the counter, which she had just been using to clean the sink, and doused her in it – through her hair, her clothes, and onto her face. He had thrown the bottle to her side once it was empty, grabbed his keys and walked out of the house locking her inside.

On hearing all this information, I strongly advised that she and her son should come up to the hospital to be checked over, and a thorough assessment of her son could be carried out to make sure there was no injuries. Unfortunately, she didn't want to come, she just wanted to be somewhere safe with her son and felt hospital wasn't where she needed to be. As a service, we can't force anyone to go to hospital if they have the mental capacity to make their own decisions, and she most certainly did.

We finished off our checks and paperwork, gave her a number for a domestic abuse helpline and finished off by asking if we could refer her child for safeguarding concerns against the partner, to which she agreed. I believed, considering the circumstances, she would understand that this would not reflect on her parenting skills and that she would regard her child's safety as paramount.

She thanked us kindly for all our help (even though we didn't do much) and we left. Walking back to the truck after hearing and seeing all of this, and having, realistically, done nothing to improve the situation, was completely draining. We hoped that we had given her some comfort and support while we were there, but this is the sad reality of this game. We are never there long enough to see the long-term changes and to help make long-term changes for the better. We are a quick band-aid fix on a mountain of problems, and sometimes that is a bitter pill to swallow.

One old mentor described this job to me one day: 'We are a jack of all trades but a master of none.' I couldn't agree more. We turn up to each job with no realistic idea as to what we are walking into, but we must be prepared for anything, so we are the jack of all trades when it comes to medicine – but no one person could have a complete knowledge of every condition, every disease, every medication and every cell in the body, so it's pretty near impossible to be a master paramedic. There are a few that probably think they're close, but that's a different story.

One of the skills that we paramedics develop over time is the ability to turn into a counsellor and social worker. Bear in mind that this is never taught to us throughout our degree: it is learned from life experience and, essentially, 'winging it'. It is probably a scary thought that a woman or man just like yourself could rock up to a person, on the worst day of their life, and it's your job to say all the right things and make everything better – and to be honest, I would completely agree. During my training I attended a woman who had tried to hang herself from the bathroom door that evening, with a rope she had found in her husband's shed. She had been diagnosed with a rare condition that caused her muscles to slowly stiffen up and soon she was going to be bed-bound. She was 45 years old and she was going blind. Her eyesight had started to deteriorate a year earlier and was now nearly completely gone. She had become solely reliant on her husband and had explained in a letter that her husband deserved to have a happy fulfilling life without her as a burden, so she had decided to take her own life to set him free.

Her husband had come home from the shops to hear banging from upstairs in the en suite bathroom. He found his wife hanging from the door nearly unconscious and blue. After swiftly cutting her down he had called 999.

When I arrived on the scene, both the patient and her husband were crying in each other's arms. This had to be the worst day of their lives and I had no idea what to say to them. 'Sorry'? 'How can I help'? 'It will be all right'? Because I knew it won't be all right – life can be bloody cruel and unforgiving and downright disgusting to good people who simply don't deserve it.

I wished more than anything I could make things better for this couple, but I couldn't. But I could offer a hand to hold, a tissue to wipe her eyes, a hug if she needed it, and an open ear to listen, which I do without hesitation.

I went home that night with a dark feeling in my chest, I remember feeling guilty for being relieved that it hadn't been me or anyone in my family. What a horrible thought to have – but it was true. I sometimes moaned that I didn't have nice hair or couldn't afford nice clothes, or that I had to study all the time and couldn't afford to go out with my friends anymore. But if I could go back to my younger self and say: 'Hey, things really aren't that bad, you could be sick or dying! A family member could be ill! You could be homeless.'

However much I might moan about being skint, I still had a roof over my head and had lived in my own flat for many years. I had been raised by a good, loving family and had amazing friends by my side. If there is one thing I will take from this job, it's never to be ungrateful or resent the things I don't have.

7

A Bailey's Too Many

One job that paramedics attend on a daily basis is DIB (difficulty in breathing) – and rightly so. Common sense tells us that if you can't breathe, you can't survive, which means that it is a life-threatening emergency that justifies calling an ambulance. Common sense would also tell you that anyone calling for an ambulance claiming DIB must be on the brink of death or at least on the road to it, but this is not the case. A lot of the time, the DIB is in fact a cough or sore throat, or a drink has gone down the wrong hole. What I have learned throughout my time is never to take what comes through on the call as gospel, because what you are expecting to find – and what you actually get – is almost always vastly different. For example, I'll give you two jobs that came through with similar descriptions but which resulted in completely different outcomes.

In the first case, we were called to a 38-year-old woman who, according to her boyfriend, was having an allergic reaction. She had had an anaphylactic attack in response to Baileys Irish Cream when she was a teenager but had decided all these years later to give it another go. (Personally, I'd say that Baileys is quite nice on the rocks, but not nice enough to risk my life for the second time.)

En route we didn't know about this previous attack, just that we were heading to another DIB/swollen face/anaphylaxis? The computer was bang on the money this time. The poor woman had managed to crawl out of her house to the front lawn in the dead of night in search of help, as she really couldn't breathe: her wheezing was audible from the confinement of the truck. Her face was so swollen I could barely distinguish her eyes from her mouth. Her skin colour was a mismatch of blue tinges and red blotches. She was in a bad way and needed help quickly.

A fast response car arrived on the scene shortly afterward and helped us immediately. She was given a concoction of a salbutamol nebuliser (in the hope of opening up her constricting airways), IM adrenaline (to help her body's response to the reaction), IV chlorphenamine (to reduce the swelling and irritation) and high flow oxygen. She was severely unstable and remained that way throughout treatment and the time in getting her to hospital. When I asked her partner how much she drank he said she had barely taken a sip before starting to complain about her throat feeling tight.

Having a severe allergy to something must be terrifying: the fear was written all over her face but I found her exhaustion more terrifying. A patient who is suffering with DIB can very quickly become exhausted and this is when things start going horribly wrong. Imagine using every possible muscle and all the strength you have just to keep breathing. Just to stay alive. I remember looking at this woman when we arrived and the panic that set off in my veins. I froze for a second (that felt like an hour) just racking my brain about what I needed to do for this woman, and the realisation came quickly that she was 'big sick'.

With a patient like this, you just want everyone and anyone to turn up and help you out, because the thought of the woman's life being in your hands for even a minute is far too long. But that's the job. Now I can't say for sure that this woman was successfully discharged from hospital: I would like to say she would probably have made a full recovery and learned to stay off the Baileys. However, you never know.

Allergic reactions aren't a new condition that most of the general public don't know about. Nonetheless, there are different stages and degrees of allergic reaction that people can get confused by, especially if someone isn't known to have an allergy. For example, there are two phases that can happen: Uniphasic is the phase which our patient in this case was experiencing. This is where the symptoms come on quickly and get rapidly worse, but once treated appropriately the symptoms resolve and usually don't return. Biphasic is when the symptoms appear mild to severe but can appear more gradually, and once treated can recur.

This is why our medical opinion for anyone that has had a bad allergic reaction is to go into the hospital for observation, or at least to stay with someone who can watch and look after you in case the symptoms recur. Nevertheless, a severe allergic reaction (anaphylaxis) always needs an immediate emergency response, as this condition can affect not just one but multiple systems of the body, from airways, heart, circulation and stomach (gut) to the skin.

8

But You Are Breathing

So, this is the second DIB/anaphylaxis job. This job came to us as a referral from 111, 111 is a non-urgent care line you can ring for advice, like 'Where is the nearest walk-in centre?' 'Can I take this medication if I'm pregnant?' Despite the great idea behind this system a lot of calls get referred to us and sometimes for the most bizarre reasons. I'll dip into that a little more later. This lady in particular had called 111 to say that her hair dye had caused her face to swell and what should she do? Granted, she should seek medical attention as I previously stated because symptoms can worsen over time. En route to this job it goes from being a CAT2 (meaning a category two) to a CAT1. Quick breakdown for you: category four is the lowest job on our scales; this means the job is not life-threatening, and going up the scale to category one – which is life-threatening with potentially imminent death. So, the description of the job had changed; this woman could no longer breathe. Her airways must have swollen and constricted so much she was no longer able to sufficiently fill her lungs. An image of the last patient is in my mind, grasping for breath, unable to stand, turning blue? We arrived on the scene at the same time as the FRC (fast response car) that was dispatched to CAT1 to aid with the life-threatening condition. We get to the door of the property for this 23-year-old female and pray that she can open the door as it is locked. After a few bangs on the door, she opens it.

'Hello, erm are we here for you?' I ask in the most non-patronising way I can. She is a healthy-looking young woman, no swelling (that I can see) breathing is perfect, good clear chest rise and no obvious DIB.

'Yeah, you're for me, come in, I put this hair dye on two days ago and now the right side of my face is swelling.' I look at her face while my colleague checks her vital signs.

'I can't see any swelling, has the swelling gone down or is it as bad as you first noticed?'

'No – it's getting worse – LOOK!' I look closer and still cannot see any difference to her face.

'OK any other symptoms? Have you got a rash anywhere? Is there any burning or itching?'

'Yes – I can't breathe.' I have issues with this statement, this is true, and I try my best to be unbiased, empathic and understanding to all patients, but in spite of that when I see patients who can quite clearly breathe compared to those who can't, it can be quite frustrating – to say the least. This lady had a clear chest of auscultation (listening), good equal chest rise and 100% oxygen levels in the blood. So, I investigate further.

'Why do you feel you can't breathe?'

'Look at me...' She waves her hand along her body like displaying a new fancy car.

I look her up and down and then back to her eye line

without making a sound. Fully aware I'm probably reeking with sarcasm but I am trying my absolute best to stay professional.

'OK Sally, when did you first notice these symptoms?'

'Yesterday before I went to bed.'

'OK, have you taken any antihistamines?'

'Yes, I got some off a friend.'

'And have they helped at all?'

'No obviously not, my face is still swollen and I can't breathe!'

'OK Sally, I'm not too sure why you feel like you cannot breathe as you are not showing any signs of someone that is having difficulty in breathing, your oxygen levels are perfect, your chest is clear, you're speaking in full clear sentences, your skin is a good healthy colour, there is no swelling to your mouth or tongue and you're able to swallow effectively as I saw you have some of your water...'

'OK well are you going to take me to hospital then?'

'Do you want to go to hospital today Sally?'

'Yes, well I think I should be seen as I'm having an allergic reaction. Where are we going to as I need to let my boyfriend know as he is driving up to meet me.'

'Where is your boyfriend now?'

'Downstairs in the car.'

'Sally, why didn't you get in your boyfriend's car and go up to the local A&E (which is 1.3 miles away) when you woke up and noticed the symptoms (which was five hours earlier)?'

'I don't know.'

'Do you want to make your way with him now? I don't feel it's necessary for you to come in the ambulance today if your boyfriend is just outside ready to take you there.'

'Well, I can't wait around there all day, I have things to do and I'll be seen quicker with you guys...' This statement is said far too much and it makes my blood boil.

'No, unfortunately not Sally, the hospital still triages the same way regardless if you're brought in by us or not.'

'Well, how long will I be up there?'

'I really can't say, maybe a couple of hours.'

'Ah no, I can't do that, maybe I'll just see how I get on.'

'Sally you've just been stating you cannot breathe to us – if you feel like that, then you should probably be in hospital.'

'Nah I feel fine now, I'll just go up later if I need to, thank you.' She gets onto the phone to her boyfriend to explain to him that her severe allergic reaction has died down and she can now breathe and that they are going to be staying at home.

'OK Sally, you have a nice day, and call us back if you are in need of an ambulance.'

We leave Sally and her boyfriend to carry out their day. This is not directly related to this patient however the emergency ambulance service is abused on a daily basis; we can be used as a taxi service, out of hours GP (even though we state on a daily basis we are not doctors), prescribers of antibiotics (which we don't do). A removal service when people don't want to look after their elderly relatives anymore. And yes, I've even been called out to clean someone's home before – actually a couple of times. I have been called out to turn off a light switch because the patient was too unwell to get out of bed and do it for themselves. It is not ideal – but what can we do, we are a free public service and often we are not allowed to say 'NO'.

9

Breathe With Me Now

Enough of the negativity for now; do you remember when I said that in my first ten weeks of training that I saw some of my sickest patients? Well, here is another example: 78-year-old Frederick. This gentleman was suffering from COPD (chronic obstructive pulmonary disease) – it is a horrendous condition that causes the lungs to become inflamed, damaged and narrowed making it increasingly difficult to breathe. It is a condition that is mostly caused by long-term smoking and which can get worse over time. Seeing a patient suffering with an exacerbation of COPD, essentially an attack, can be a terrifying thing for the clinician and patient because they simply can't get the air into their lungs to breathe. Their lungs have become so constricted and narrowed that air won't go in.

Well, that is exactly what was happening for this gentleman – he was having an attack and a bad one. His home contained every piece of evidence that this gentleman had breathing problems: his bed was propped up by three or four pillows because he could no longer sleep on his back; he had a CPAP machine (that helps force air into the lungs when he was sleeping); and the classic dirty ashtray lying next to his bed. For the life of me I still can't understand why the appeal of smoking would still exist when every time you smoke one you must feel like you're dying, but people still do every day. His wife answered the door with a concerned look on her face.

This first greeting with a family member tells the crew a lot. If they look scared then we have a job on our hands. We walked in to see Frederick sitting bolt upright on his bed, hands on his knees, using every muscle in his body to gasp even a fraction of air. He was wearing his CPAP machine also, but this wasn't helping at all. I was only a few weeks into training and I quickly looked at my mentor for guidance while connecting him up to our life pack to check his vital signs. His oxygen levels were low, very low. This meant he wasn't breathing in enough oxygen to perform a gas exchange within the lungs and get oxygen into the blood to perfuse the body.

This means the brain is being starved of oxygen, which is called hypoxia. This can cause confusion, irritation, aggression, and even death. We immediately started acting on a treatment plan – he needed oxygen and salbutamol to try and open up his airways, from the very base of his lungs you could hear a faint wheezing. This was enough for us to try a neb (nebuliser) to see if this helped. When I trained, we could apply a nebuliser to a bag valve mask through a T-piece. This basically means we could fill a bag full of oxygen and the steamed salbutamol together, and when we pressed hard on the bag it would force itself into his lungs. It is a lot like the CPAP machine.

My mentor asked me to bag the patient while she sorted out an extraction plan. When I placed the mask over his face with my hands shaking, the patient grabbed hold of me and my hands and said 'Please – I can't breathe,' in broken gasps of air. I pressed hard on the bag and oxygen forced its way into his body, but there was resistance as he was trying to breathe on his own.

'OK Sir, when I say breathe take a deep breath in and I'll press the bag. We're going to need to do this together.'

'BREATHE', I pressed the bag again and the oxygen went in and I saw his chest rise properly for the first time. He was still panicking, though, and squeezed my hands tighter and tighter.

'BREATHE.' He took another large gasp in and again I saw his chest rising and falling.

'Qui-ck-er,' he managed to say one broken word but I know what he meant.

'OK – BREATHE… BREATHE… BREATHE.' His wife was looking on in horror as a young 20-something-year-old that she had never met before, clearly scared out of her mind, did the breathing for her husband. His oxygen levels were only improving slightly, while my mentor and another crew member from the truck were busy sorting out other things… what things, I don't know to this day, because the whole time I didn't break eye contact with this man.

Our breathing even synced. When he breathed, I breathed. He held onto my hands so he was holding the mask and the bag as if we were doing it together. *Please God don't die,* I thought. I had stages in my head, and I think a lot of clinicians will work this way when someone is big sick: if we can get the patient off the bed and onto a chair alive, that's one stage done… now let's get him out of the house… now let's get him on the bed in the truck, reconnect him to the machines there, put a blue call in and be ready to bomb it to hospital… get to hospital…

hand over to the staff there. Each of these stages are individual jobs aimed at keeping the patient alive. Keep him breathing and raise his oxygen levels – or at least don't let them fall any more at each stage – and we could get him to the hospital alive.

So that is what I did.

'BREATHE... BREATHE...' While my mentors were managing the amount of oxygen that he was having due to being a COPD patient (they unfortunately can't be flooded with oxygen as this can have an adverse effect), I was none the wiser at this stage of my training. So, I stuck to my patient like glue and we continued to breathe together. We got him into hospital and were about to carry out the last stage: handover. Now I can't say what my mentor's and colleagues' faces looked like, but I'm sure mine was a sweaty, flushed, nervous mess with pleading eyes that said: *Help me. I'm way out of my depth here.*

The staff quickly took a handover and started treating the patient. We packed up our kit and left after the paperwork was done. My mentor thanked me for my hard work, something I felt awkward for accepting, and then decided to sit in silence for the remainder of the time until the next job came in.

It is safe to say that from this point onwards, when DIB came down on the ambulance computer, I would shit myself a tiny bit.

10

Help Please, I Don't Know What I'm Doing

U sually when someone of a young age, let's say below 50, calls with chest pain, they have a far lower chance of having a real cardiac issue like a heart attack. Now that's not to say that they aren't experiencing pain. However, I wouldn't be wrong to be thinking in terms of differential diagnoses while en route to these patients. So, when we got a call to a young 19-year-old male in his student accommodation at midnight on a Wednesday, my first thought wasn't cardiac. The thoughts going through my mind were: *Chest infection? Anxiety? Trauma? Muscular pain?*

Without a proper examination and vital signs check I could have thrown a hundred differential diagnoses out there, but we would never know until we had seen him ourselves. We arrived at the student housing where a reception/security guard had no idea of our expected arrival and asked us worriedly what room we were meant to be going to.

'Room 42, could you show us where we are going?'

'Yes of course, come this way.'

'Help help – he's up here!' A young lad was shouting, waving at us from the lift lobby.

'Ahh never mind, thank you Sir, we can follow him.' I noticed the worried expression on his face. Again, you ask yourself a series of questions: is this friend over-worrying, adrenaline-filled because an ambulance is about to attend his friend or is our patient going to be big sick? What I did notice, getting a little side-tracked on my way up, was that this was NICE student housing, nothing like mine. It had white marble flooring, plants all over the place, and fancy art, and cleanliness just poured out of this place.

If you had swabbed some of the houses based around my University you would have been able to identify three new species never seen before! The young lad was in his sportswear, as if he had just come back from a midnight workout after a busy day's studying. Or else it could just be the normal attire for these young students. He pushed the number three in the lift several times in the hope it would make the lift move faster, but of course it didn't. We all know this, but it did remind me of something that might happen in a movie.

'Can you tell me what's happened to your friend then?'

'I don't know, he was with his girlfriend in his room and then she came out banged on my door and was screaming that he needed help, so I called you guys – but he looks in a bad way!' I glanced at my mentor with a suspicious look of wonder, meaning: *I think this guy is going to be big sick, you know.*

We went into his room and another surprise was that each student had their own apartment, and not just a box room big enough to fit a single bed. This one had a huge desk, a double bed, and a little kitchen fitted at the back. This place was insane.

Another more crucial thing I noticed was the man lying on the floor drenched in sweat, clutching his chest as if to stop his heart from bursting out. He was pale white from the torso down, but an odd shade of purple/red from the shoulders up. If we were in a WWF fight right now, this is where I would tap out and let someone else take over, because he looked big sick and I knew I had no clue what was wrong with him.

Being a first-year student really did suck in that way: I wanted nothing more than to swoop in and act quickly like the rest of the crew – with a grace and calm that showed they knew exactly what they were doing. I just kept telling myself that in time I would be like them and not this fumbling mess playing dress-up.

The crew started treating him – his oxygen levels were low for someone of his health and build, and his heart rate was reaching the high 130's, which wasn't surprising given the amount of pain he appeared to be in. He had just been lying in bed with his girlfriend and out of nowhere this pain had smacked him in the chest. We blued him into hospital of course, but on the way down from his room the whole dorm had apparently got word of what had been happening on the third floor, so now there was a herd of students waiting in the common room downstairs with video cameras, filming our departure and shouting well wishes as we left. It felt a bit like a parade but, hey that was their way of saying goodbye, I guess.

The young lad would have been fine after his stint in the hospital. After being diagnosed with a massive pulmonary embolism in his lung he was treated accordingly. But this poor lad was 19 years old. To have such a serious medical condition hit him out of nowhere really does prove that no one is safe.

THE FIRST YEAR DONE

After a few nights out drinking and hugs goodbye, I had completed my first year as a student paramedic. My Mum was so proud and, to be honest, so was I! But it still didn't feel real – it felt as if I was on work experience and that it would be over soon, and I would be back to my normal nine-to-five. The prospect of me actually becoming a paramedic didn't really sink in until the third year.

I didn't really live the party lifestyle in my first couple of years at University. I would like to say that it was because I was studying hard all the time, but the truth was that I lived far from the University and I was (and still am) a pretty shy, anxious person. I wish I could make friends easily but I would sit on my own in the lecture rooms and keep myself to myself. I made one friend during my induction and we would sit together and meet for lectures. She left during the second year.

I always got it into my head that people wouldn't want me to sit with them or join their group. I would make up scenarios in my head, thinking that they would look and talk about me, saying things like: 'Why is she joining us?'; 'Who is this girl?' Of course, they probably wouldn't have done that, but I couldn't shake that feeling, so to save myself the anxiety I would just keep myself to myself.

That is why, when group scenarios or group activities came up, I would shrivel into a ball and hope no one noticed that I didn't put myself into a group. I hated acting in front of the class and being the lead clinician in case I did something wrong and people judged me or laughed at me.

In reality, everyone was in the same boat and probably knew just as little as I did! I would be jealous of the loud pack-leaders of the class who had a gang of friends around them cracking jokes and who were always running the scenarios because they had the confidence to do it.

To this day I am extremely proud of myself for sticking it out, as there were so many times I just wanted to go home, shut my door to the world and choose an easier life. But in my heart, I knew it wasn't my inability to do the job that was holding me back: it was simply my confidence.

I kept telling myself that confidence would come in time, and I suppose in the end it did!

II

Second Year Student Paramedic

11

Mental Health On The Road

My second year flew by, it seemed like it was over before it had started. This was the year when I knew a lot more and was able to do much more with respect to treating and managing patients, but still didn't have the responsibility and realisation that would come from knowing I was nearly qualified, so this was the most laid-back year in my eyes. Which is the wrong approach, I know.

I got an insight into the reality of mental health and its failings, I saw my first CVA (stroke), my first cardiac arrest and my first shooting. Again, these are the jobs that stuck with me. I was put at a different station this time round: it was smaller, with a tight-knit group who worked there. I was seriously intimidated when I first walked in, but soon realised that everyone was lovely and welcoming, and liked to have a laugh.

MENTAL HEALTH ON THE ROAD

The subject of mental health covers such a mixture of conditions and diagnoses, that it would take a degree in itself to fully understand the ins and out of each condition and how to react and treat each one. I already mentioned what one of my mentors said: 'We are jack of all trades, but master of none.' And this is so true. We try our very best to understand and learn and treat, but we don't always know the answers and will sometimes have to ask the patient what their condition means and how it affects them. When it comes to mental health there are so many rules and what I like to call 'by-laws' that we must follow.

For example: you cannot take someone to hospital against their will if they lack the capacity to make a decision due to their mental health. However, if they are a danger to themselves or others you can make a request to the police to section them. This all depends whether they are in their home or out in public. We can get a patient sectioned under a section 2, which means a doctor will come and assess the patient and see if they need admitting to a ward.

I have spent many hours on the scene with a patient trying to inform them that hospital would be good for them and they are having a crisis: it leaves ambulance staff in a horrible position when someone clearly needs some help – but they can't see why they need help due to their condition. My management plan when I started would have been hospital every time, but I soon realised through studies and research that actually hospitalising someone for a crisis or an acute episode of mental health isn't always beneficial. It often leads to their condition worsening, because the patient is led to believe that they are going to become 'all better' but actually leave the hospital feeling no different. Which negatively affects their mental health even more!

The crisis teams, helplines and charities that work for people with these conditions are great! I have always had a good experience with mental health teams – they often know the patient on a first-name basis and know how to calm them down and talk to them on a personal level, which I may not be able to do having only known them for around 30 minutes. This often leads to the patient not needing to go into hospital, or the crisis team coming out to visit them that day to chat properly. This will always be my first line of treatment before heading off to hospital as I have seen far better plans come together when I have left the patient at home, and I really feel it was often in the patient's best interest. At the end of the day, we are here to *help* people and not just be a shiny yellow taxi to the hospital. If we can relieve the stress in A&E and treat patients at home, then it's been a good day in my books.

There is still a stigma to mental illness. Some will say: 'But I'm not crazy' if you mention mental health, depression or anxiety. Having a mental health condition doesn't make you crazy! It is a disorder that can be treated in a variety of ways from simply having a conversation to medication. Everyone has different levels and different treatment plans.

I think we all have some kinds of mental health issues that develop throughout our lives – and that's just called living in my opinion. According to the charity MIND, one in four people have a mental health problem in any given year! One in six people will suffer with anxiety or depression in any given week. Suicide is on the rise and factors such as money, jobs and social media have strong effects on mental health.

Mental health awareness isn't just about the people with diagnosed mental disorders that need to be either hospitalised or heavily treated: it's also about the common day-to-day living that we all experience. And let's be honest, we all need a little help from time to time. I can't count the number of times I have opened my phone and gone on social media only to shut it down as my anxiety became too heavy on my chest. The reasons why this has happened I still don't truly understand.

In a survey carried out in the UK in 2016, anxiety and depression were ranked the most common mental health problems. This is why we attend people with these symptoms so often on the ambulance. Someone may be OK one minute, then the next they are having a raging panic attack, can't control their breathing, and, no matter how hard they try, they can't seem to get it under control. This makes a lot of people think they are dying. When I recognise this is happening to one of my patients, then my yoga voice comes out! I tell them everything will be OK and to control their breathing. I tell them to hold their breath between each exhalation.

I learned this from watching my mentors in the second year. It takes a while to settle everything down, but it does work. At the end of the day, the patient is in a state of panic, so calming them down and slowing everything down is essential.

12

Know Your FAST Symptoms

This job stuck with me because, when we arrived on the scene, the patient was a happy chippy 50-year-old man heading off to sunny Tenerife the next day with his wife for their anniversary. He hadn't wanted to make a fuss and didn't want an ambulance, but his wife had insisted and now he appeared to be getting worse. Up to this point I had never seen a stroke before, I had seen the adverts about FAST and the typical facial drop. But had never witnessed it happening first-hand. It is key to remember that strokes do not always present with the typical FAST symptoms: things can catch you off guard and simple leg pain can turn out to be something a lot worse.

'So, what's happened this morning Jerry?'

'I got up in the night to go for a piss, excuse me... use the toilet, and as I got up my left leg went. I fell to the floor and it took a while to get me back up, then I kind of dragged to the toilet, done me business then went back to bed... woke up this morning and it's a bit better but still not right.'

'He can barely walk and when he does, he's all over the place.'

His wife sounded concerned.

'OK, does it hurt at all?'

'Nah, not a bit: just feels funny, almost like it's not my leg.' At this point we were all thinking there was probably a neurological cause, but what it could be we were unsure. I quickly performed a FAST test and it was only failing on his leg. His hand strength was great – he nearly broke my fingers! – and his smile was perfect. So, we were all scratching our heads. Nonetheless, it needed to be checked out, so off we popped to hospital. They lived on the 14th floor, so I asked my colleague if he wouldn't mind grabbing the chair. At that, Jerry stood up, looking kind of wobbly, and said: 'Don't be silly. I'm not going in a chair. I can make my way.'

'Oh, Jerry let them do their job and take you on the chair!'

'Yes, honestly, Jerry. We don't mind, I'd rather you were comfortable rather than trying to make your way down the stairs.'

'No – I'm fine, I can walk, thank you, my dear, I'm not dying yet!' He laughed off his shaking leg, and I remember laughing too. We held his arms as we made our way to the lift. Once in the lift he began to put more weight onto us and I asked repeatedly if he was OK. His response was slow and I began to panic. Something wasn't right. Once we were out of the lift, he could barely hold himself upright and my mentor shouted at his crewmate to get the chair back ASAP. I tried to get an answer out of my patient and he was grumbling words out that made no real sense. He was still fully conscious but couldn't form words to express what he was saying.

We all knew what was happening. He was having a massive stroke. We got him into the ambulance as quickly as possible and blue lighted him to the nearest HASU centre (which is where stroke patients go). By the time we had arrived at the hospital and handed over our patient, he couldn't speak and had lost a lot of motor function. I was in disbelief. Just 20 minutes earlier, he had been drinking his morning cuppa and telling me about his morning piss!

We hung around to find out what happened. When we were told that he had had a massive bleed on the brain (known as a haemorrhagic stroke), it was gut-wrenching. He had lost most motor function and speech. The doctor's diagnosis was he would probably be bed-bound after this.

I couldn't look at his wife; I was in shock myself, so how his wife must have felt was beyond belief. How can life change so quickly, so cruelly and without warning? And again, there are the inevitable questions: Would that have happened if we had insisted on the chair? Could we have been quicker? What if he had called during the night when it first happened?

There have been many times in my short career when I have questioned myself as to whether I could have done something differently, made a better decision, or chosen a different path. I imagine I will have many more such times to come, but I do have to remind myself that, no matter how good it is to question and continually improve yourself, I can't beat myself up over decisions I have made because I know in my heart that at that time and place, I was doing my absolute best for my patient and nothing I do now can change that. I can only change things for the better in the future. So, I will study and learn until I decide this job is no longer for me, or I retire, and at this rate that will be when I'm 75.

13

Paediatrics

I can't say I know many paramedics that don't have paediatrics as their horror jobs, meaning the jobs that they pray they don't get. I remember naively saying as a student that I didn't mind paediatric jobs and was happy to work them!

Firstly, I cringe at how naive and cocky that sounds; and secondly I wish I could stop myself back then and say: 'Erm… you're wrong but you will soon learn that nothing scares you more than sick children. So be prepared.' I think this fear has been slowly building, and one year after becoming a fully qualified paramedic I had a terrible job involving a 10-year-old girl, which was my personal breaking point. We will get to that little girl later on. For now, let's start with the first building block in my tower of fear.

NEGLECT AND OVERDOSES

One time, we were called to a 13-year-old male who was

unconscious. I was attending as I did every day, but this time my mentor and I were in a car doing a first responder shift. Basically, cars will go to CAT 1 jobs; back when I was a student, cars went to CAT 2 jobs as well. They were designed so paramedics or emergency ambulance-trained staff could get on the scene quickly and begin life-saving treatment while a truck was still en route. We arrived on the scene to this patient in no time and grabbed all the kit we thought we needed. After we had hauled all our bags up two flights of unlit stairs a little boy came out of a flat and said: 'You're here for my brother.'

'Ah thank you, young man, can you show me where we are going?' He led us into a dimly lit flat: well actually, it wasn't lit at all. The only light on was the bathroom light.

'Can we have some lights on please?' I asked. I remember saying this because, as I did, my mentor quietly said 'well done' as they often did when I remembered key things like this.

Always go into a property with light and good access for getting back out again if we need to.

The mother came out of the room calmly and said 'No lights,' waving at the empty light socket on the ceiling. Her broken English told us that she didn't speak the language well, which could lead to difficult communication and problems in getting the medical history.

Before I explain how we found our patient, I want to add that paramedics are optimistic beings and we always hope for the best. That means we hope that the patient is in fact conscious or, if they are unconscious, that after a light pinch to the trapezius muscle their eyes will suddenly open. This is usually the case, and a lot of the time 'life-threatening' emergencies are in fact not life-threatening at all.

On this occasion, that was my thought process: he will be

awake or tired on his bed, maybe with the flu. What I was greeted with was a young boy lying on his bedroom floor in a pool of water. My mentor and I sprang into action and I immediately remembered my ABC's – I look back to this job as the one when I really started to learn and act upon what I had learnt without second guessing myself.

I tried to get a pain response from him, but he had no reaction. So, my mentor tried a lot harder and still got nothing. I opened his airway and looked down his throat with the little light I had and it appeared to be OK. Then I moved down to feel for a pulse and look at his breathing. While I was doing this my crewmate was also feeling for a radial. He had a strong bounding carotid pulse and was breathing quickly. This was a small moment of relief but it didn't last long.

'What's happened!' my mentor snapped at the mother who was at this point trying to entertain the other child and keep him occupied.

'I don't know, he wouldn't wake up. He sleeps all day.'

'All day?!' I snapped back quickly, not checking my attitude.

'When was the last time you saw him awake and talking?' my mentor asked, as she was fitting equipment.

'Around 7pm.' It was about 8pm at this point, so we had a one-hour window in which we didn't know what had happened to this boy.

'7pm yesterday…'

'Yesterday! He has been in bed since yesterday and you didn't wake him?'

'I tried but he wouldn't get up, he's a young boy and lazy.' At this point we knew a few things: his oxygen levels were low; his heart rate was slightly high and his blood pressure was on the low side of normal. Also, his sugar levels were fine so we ruled out hypoglycaemia. And one last thing which I realised – this mother, for whatever reason, was goddamn neglectful in my book!

The crew of the truck arrived and helped us carry him to the bathroom for better light. The team worked away getting lines in and giving fluids and oxygen. Once he was more stable, we started to get an extraction plan together. One of the members of staff went into the patient's room to have a look around for any sign as to what had caused this and found a bottle of liquid paracetamol lying empty in his bed. He asked the mother if this was his and whether it was a new bottle. She replied it was a new bottle, so now we were looking at a paracetamol overdose as the main diagnosis, and one that had progressively got worse over the course of 24 hours.

On the way to the hospital, he was on his own with us, as his mother chose to go up to the hospital with her sister and didn't want to come in the ambulance. So, I had to get his personal details once we had arrived. I started by asking his name and date of birth. She couldn't tell me his date of birth, simply saying 'erm, I don't know.'

'What do you mean? You don't know his birthday?'

'No.' She gave me a half-confused smile, as though to say *sorry*. I asked for the other children's details, as they were in the house, and got the same answer. I still don't know if she didn't want to give them to me or whether she really didn't know her own children's birthdays. It may have been a religious belief not to celebrate birthdays, or the dates had simply got lost in her memory. However, it was a bitter pill for me to swallow.

We later found out that he had indeed consumed the entire bottle and slipped into a coma due to the toxins in his liver entering his bloodstream and causing his brain to swell.

I never found out if he recovered, I can only hope.

My mother is the light of my life. It was she who guided me and taught me to be the person I am. Don't get me wrong – my Dad has shown me strength, loyalty, honesty and love. But the bond I have developed with my Mum is special. We are two sides of a whole: apart we're OK, but when we're together, it's pretty fucking awesome. She has cared for me and loved me since the day I was born, and to make her proud is one of my biggest goals in life.

She has some amazing quirks that used to annoy me when I was younger but which I now find hilarious! She is paranoid about everything when it comes to her children's safety. We were put in brightly coloured clothing so we could easily be spotted in a crowd. I was never allowed more than two feet away from her in public, right up until I was about 15 years old. She still goes to grab my hand when we're crossing a road, at the age of 29. Also, she has me on Tracker so she can see where I am and when I'm home! That is where she wants me to be.

I recently found out after I had returned from a holiday in Mexico that on the day after I had flown out, she had broken down in tears at work because I was too far away. She also has this weird ability to know when something isn't right with me. Now, I'm not saying she can tell when I'm down, because most people can do that: I'm a pretty open book. But she can tell if I'm in trouble.

Listen to this and tell me there isn't something weird going on... I had left my car at a pub after having deciding to have a drink and taking a cab home. Next morning, I asked if my Mum could drop me at my car, which she kindly agreed to do. We chatted away and when we arrived at my car, we hugged and said our goodbyes.

I got into my car after she had driven off and started heading out myself. However, I noticed two minutes into my drive that the car was feeling awful and something wasn't right. By this point though, I was on a winding country road with nowhere to pull over. So, I chugged along until I saw a turning down a single lane track that led to a care home. Once I was around the corner, the lane was completely hidden by hedges, so I was now hidden, out of sight from the road. I had NO signal on my phone, because we live in the ass end of nowhere, and I had a completely flat tire with no spare. GREAT.

I pondered my options for a few minutes and decided all I could do is walk home, which is about 40 minutes: or at least walk until I had a signal and could call for help. I started walking back down the driveway and my Mum's car pulled in!

'What the hell, how did you know I was here!'

'I knew it, I knew something was wrong so I turned around. When I couldn't see your car up to this point, I thought you might have turned in here to get off the road.'

'What do you mean, you knew something was wrong?'

'I just knew.'

Now, I know that every family is different and every mother is different. Personally, I am a Step-mummy to a beautiful little boy and Mummy to my fur baby, and I have definitely inherited my Mum's overprotectiveness: I'm always saying: 'Oh no, he can't do that or this could happen...' But in my head, that's what Mums do – they protect their babies, no matter how old they are. That is why I find it so hard when I go to some patients who are babies themselves, and their Mum seems to know so little about what's going on. I have had three really sick children in my years on the road, cases where I have thought: *Wow – this could be it; they might die here.* And for two of them, the Mums spent their time texting on the phone instead of holding their child's hand or screaming at me to know if their child was OK.

This is what I expect, this is what I prepare for. Everyone deals with stress differently. But I had one Mum ask me if she was OK to leave (go home) when we were standing in resus with about ten hospital staff around her child, fighting to keep her alive.

Whether it was my place to say it or not I said: 'No, your child is very sick and she needs you here. You're staying!' At this point I had to walk off to catch my breath and calm down.

As we are on the subject of children, I will tell you next about my first shooting.

And yes, a child was shot.

14

Bruv I Got Shot

We were called to a 13-year-old female, who had been shot in the back in a drive-by shooting that had clearly gone wrong. I mean drive by shootings can't exactly go right, but you get what I mean. We were slightly confused, as the address given was outside a police station. Surely no one would actually shoot someone in the police station, so we wondered if they had been brought there for safety.

When we arrived on the scene, it looked like something out of a movie. The front of the police station was taped off, with police standing guard all around. Just by the front steps to the entrances there was a black car, half on the pavement and half with its nose smashed up against someone else's car. In the back of the car along the rear there were three or four clear bullet holes dotted around the boot. We went quickly into the police station to find our patient, who we were told was sitting in one of the side meeting rooms chatting away with the police officers.

This is when your hopeful mind heaves a big sigh of relief! We got into see her and the officer had been right – she was sitting bent over laughing and giggling with the officer in the room.

'Hello there!'

'Oh hi, so I guess you're here for me? I'm fine. I think I was shot in the back?'

'Erm, well let's hope not... you don't look like someone that was shot to me!'

I had a quick look at her back and she did indeed have a small circular laceration, almost like a burn mark on her back. It was superficial and had barely broke through the deep layers of tissue. It was incredible: I was wondering how the bullet had stopped just enough to break the outer surfaces of the skin but nothing else.

Once everything appeared to be OK with our patient, we had a chat to the police officer, and he told us that there was a large tub of protein mix (gym powder, I call it) in the boot of the car, and the bullet had gone through that. So, it had acted like a sandbag and slowed the bullet down. I was speechless. . .PROTEIN SHAKE, the most annoying product ever to be splattered all over Instagram and Facebook had just saved this little girl's life!

We transported her to hospital and this is where we got an insight into the life that this little girl led. Her phone rings.

'Yoooo bruv, you'll never guess what's just happened, I GOT SHOT bruv.'

'I know can't fucking believe it, nah I'm cool man.'

'Just my back fucking hurts!'

'Drive-by yeah!'

'Fucking insane man.' Then she continued to post the riveting tale on her Snapchat.

I'm at a loss for words.

15

My First Cardiac Arrest

Everyone remembers their first cardiac arrest. Mine didn't come down the line as a cardiac arrest. It came down as DIB choking, and I believe this was what was happening before she stopped breathing. When we arrived, our motorbike responder was already on the scene doing CPR, and they had the defibrillator attached. I felt a surge of adrenaline rise from my feet to my head and my hands began to shake and sweat.

'Shall I jump on the chest?' (Not literally.)

'Yes please.'

My mentor stepped in: 'Em, you need airways signing off so get on the airway.'

'OK...' I moved over towards the patient's head and began to size up equipment, and my crewmate helped get all the kit out. Thank God he was there, as I would have flapped and not really known what I was looking for, or how to set things up properly! There is a certain way all the pieces of the airway kit fit together, and when in a panic there is nothing worse than trying to thumb together an airway tube. He did it quickly and panic-free, like it was second nature, and handed me all the kit. I began to look into the airway and make sure there was nothing that would block the trachea. It looked all clear so I fitted an I-GEL Supraglottic airway. It went in first time and I was surprised at the clear chest rise I was getting when bagging. It was in, it's working well!

'Well done Em, now jump on the chest.' You get told horror stories about CPR, especially about bones cracking. If there is one thing that I can't stand, it's deformed bones and the sound of them breaking. So, the idea of breaking them with my hands and feeling them shatter makes my skin crawl. Because I wasn't the first person doing CPR, I didn't feel any bones break and that was a small relief.

Not too long had passed and there were six members of staff there, including an advanced paramedic. They're basically the boss when they arrive on the scene and they will take control and tell us what to do, and you know what – I'm completely fine with that!

We worked on this lady, who was probably only 50 at the time, for a while. Her rhythms kept changing and we weren't sure if we could get her back. We ended up taking her to hospital while still actively working a resus. I was asked to continue CPR in the truck as we drove on blue lights to the hospital.

As you can imagine it was extremely difficult and tiring but that's not what was going through my head at the time. I was thinking: *how the hell did I get here? I went from replying to emails and writing cover letters in an office to 'jumping' up and down on someone's chest in the middle of the night while in a moving van that's probably travelling at 30 mph through central London!*

We didn't get this lady back – she was declared dead shortly after our arrival at hospital, with her family by her side.

Coming to the end of my second year of University and my confidence was high, while my emotions were good. I was feeling positive about work. The year of dissertations and final exams had begun. All that was in my path before qualifying was a few grades and my last ten-week placement.

On the first day of my last placement, it hit me that this would be the last time I was on the road as a student. After those ten weeks I would be doing the job like my mentors. Registered and fully liable for anything and everything that happens to my patients. No room for mistakes. It is surprising how quickly ten weeks can pass when you don't actually want them to be over. I wanted to be paid for my work, granted, but the idea of all that responsibility hit me hard and the panic set in. I was thinking: *Am I ready for all this? Can I make these decisions all on my own?*

I still didn't grasp the true reality of this job even in my last year of placement. You are still being guided and taught, even up to your last day. Also, some mentors are more forward in their teaching. Some will push you to make a decision to see if you actually can, and others will just let you sit in the background and then sign your portfolio off to say you did that job when really you didn't: it makes an easier life for themselves.

I didn't enjoy my time with these mentors because I wondered what I was really learning? I could watch and learn but there's nothing better for me than using my brain and coming up with a solution that everyone else agrees with. Then I feel successful and my confidence grows. I had a few mentors along the way that taught me many insightful things and there were some that taught me how *not* to practice medicine. Either way

I was learning.

I was beginning to make friends too, which I was overjoyed about. However, I still wasn't confident enough to join them when they asked me out for after work drinks. I didn't feel I could, as I was just a student. Not a fully accepted member of staff. I was older than some of the qualified medics but I felt like a young child compared to them and I really don't know why.

III

Third Year Student Paramedic

Final Year of Education

16

Feeling Better Now Are We?

I have been to a lot of jobs now which involve either the police or the courts where the patient has requested us as they are feeling unwell. Now I can't say for certain that the patient isn't telling the whole truth about their symptoms, but you often wonder if they have asked for us in order to get themselves out of the jam that they're in.

Just because you go to hospital doesn't mean that the laws you have broken will automatically go away. So again, I'm not sure why people do this – but they do. Someone will get caught shoplifting and when caught suddenly lose consciousness and come over feeling unwell. They always regain consciousness when we arrive. One of these jobs I remember well resulted in the patient's 'life-changing symptoms' completely resolving when a vehicle malfunction caused us to tip off the back of the ambulance. She soon moved her limbs at the prospect of face-planting the ground. To cut a long story short, this woman was picked up by us in the police station, where she was in giving a statement? Evidence? Confession? I don't know. However, at some point she became 'unwell', collapsed in the chair and wouldn't respond to the police officers.

When we arrived, the lady was wrapped up in blankets with a crowd of police officers standing over her. They looked rather concerned or at least confused. It seems that she had slumped to one side during the interview and then collapsed to the floor. The female police officer taking the interview believed she had had a stroke. We woke this woman up pretty quickly with a pinch to the shoulder. (Don't worry, this is procedure when someone is unconscious, it's called a pain stimulus.) She made out to us that she couldn't speak at all, which was the first sign something was off. When someone is having a bad stroke, you can kind of tell, straight off the bat. Granted, it isn't always obvious. I mentioned that earlier in this book, but when someone loses their speech that doesn't mean they won't try to get their words out. It either comes out slurred or muddled – I have seen it many times, where the patient is trying so hard to say something but just can't get the words out. However, this lady was shaking her hand at me to say: 'No I can't speak.'

I tried the FAST test, which is the test to help assess if someone is suffering from a stroke: a quick test to assess speech, arms, face, and leg strength. We want to see equal strength of both sides of the body, symmetrical facial movements and clear or normal speech. This lady was completely failing the FAST test, as every time I asked her to raise her arms, I would assist in lifting them and then one arm would fall immediately to the ground with a slap. She couldn't smile at all, and couldn't use one leg. Her left side appeared to have gone. There was nothing else for us to do: we had to assume this was real and took her off to the nearest stroke unit in London on blue lights. She was doubly strapped in bed and all precautions had been taken in case this was a real stroke... which my gut was telling me it wasn't. But what can I say? I'm no doctor.

When we got to hospital, we opened up the tail lift to bring the trolley bed down. As my crewmate pressed the button to lower the tail lift, I felt a jolt and suddenly the trolley bed was rolling off the end of the ambulance about two foot off the ground. I panicked and tried to hold the trolley bed on the platform with all my strength but when gravity took over, I flew over the handles of the bed and crashed onto the floor next to it. Luckily the trolley beds have poles on either side. So, the patient was strapped into the bed and the whole bed landed completely straight. I jumped up to check if the patient was OK and saw her fiercely grabbing hold of her son with both hands (with firm grips). He was standing in front of her and she was also screaming from the shock. Firstly, her voice had come back; secondly her strength had come back as could be clearly seen in the crease lines in her son's shirt. And the speech and facial movements were definitely not impaired.

'Ah thank goodness you're OK! And you seem to be moving again.'

Patient: silence.

'Are you feeling any better?'

Patient: silence.

'You can talk again – you just spoke to your son.'

Son: 'What's going on, is she OK?'

'Yes, let's get her into the hospital. I'm sure it will be OK. The doctors will look after her now.'

In my head: *She's OK but I have two busted knees! Brilliant.*

17

So Who's Going To Clean Up This Mess?

Have you ever been at work and thought: *This is not my bloody job* and become angry... you're tired and hungry and then you have some rather unsavoury person try and tell you what your job actually is? Well, I definitely have. I'll set the scene and then let's see if you understand why I was pissed off.

It was 4:30 am on the night shift, third of a run of four. We were called to an intoxicated male, in a flat, with his friends. We arrived on the scene and this fella was fast asleep in bed, next to a pretty full vomit bowl. His friends told us about their night of drinking, explaining that the male had become sick and was throwing up all over the place. They had mixed their drinks from brandy to tequila to beer and then finished it off with wine.

So not surprisingly he vomited most of it back up again. We woke up the male to see if he was OK and he apologised profusely that we had been called, saying he just needed to sleep it off. Which I completely agreed with. I mean, we've all been there so there was no judgement on my part.

Then we explained to his friends that he was medically fine and just needed to sleep it off and be in a place of safety with his friends to look out for him. He'd been asleep for about three hours and after a few more hours he would be OK. Simple.

The female friends thanked us for coming and were just happy that their friend was going to be OK. The male friend, on the other hand, was not happy with our assessment and revealed the real reason he called the emergency ambulance service.

'Look, so are you not going to take him?'

'No, he's OK and does not need to be in A&E, why?'

'Well, he has thrown up all over my flat!'

'I see that, but he's not medically very unwell and in need of treatment – he just needs to stay hydrated and sleep this off, which he can do here. He does not need a bed in A&E.'

'Look, I have work in three hours... can you just take him?!'

'Erm, no sorry, that's not how it works.'

'Right, so what about the vomit?'

'Again, that's not our job to clean that up either...' He looked completely pissed off that we had declined his polite offer to clean up the vomit from his carpet floor. Surely this guy hadn't called us firstly to take his friend off his hands just 'cause he was drunk and clearly annoying him, and secondly to clean up vomit at 4:30 in the morning?!

Safe to say we did the paperwork pretty sharpish. We checked once more that the patient was OK and happy to stay in bed and sleep it off, which he agreed to, and then we were on our way again. Back out to save another life...

18

One Under

I'll start this chapter by breaking down the title. A 'one under' means a person or persons trapped under 'something' – usually a train or a vehicle from a road traffic accident. For this particular patient it was a train – an overground train to be more precise. They gave no information on age or gender for the patient as the call came down and, yes, you'll will have guessed, I have never dealt with a 'one under' and we were also just 0.7 miles away from the incident, so we were going to be the first on the scene.

I had already undertaken my training for train safety and the procedures for this kind of job, but I still felt like I was way over my head. We pulled up at the entrance of the train station and started to collect our bags and any pieces of kit we thought we might need. So basically everything!

Just to highlight how quickly we were on the scene: passengers were still getting off the train as we were walking down to the platform. I was the first to the platform and a network rail worker standing on the platform in bright orange overalls pointed to an opening between the carriage and the tracks underneath. The workers had been there doing some repairs to the platform and parts of the platform were boarded off. I remember thinking that once I looked down this gap, I would be confronted with something horrific.

This is where things become extremely dark; if this person was still alive, they would either be in horrendous pain, or actively dying, or indeed both. Until the power is off and we get the all clear that it is safe to approach the tracks there is simply nothing we can do for the patient, and the dark side is that confirming the power is off can take a while. I looked through the gap and the patient laid over the track. His abdomen was on the tracks, indicating that the train had driven straight over his stomach. He looked grey already and completely lifeless. Without even getting near to this gentleman I could see he was dead. He was middle-aged. The person in charge of confirming power is called a RIO: I'm not sure why but that means he/she is the person you want to find on the platform to get further instructions. It must have been a few minutes but it felt as though the platform was instantly swarming with BTP (British Transport Police), LFB (London Fire Brigade), HART (Hazardous Area Response Team), HEMS (the trauma specialists I mentioned earlier) CTL (Clinical Team Leaders) and FRU (Fast Response Cars).

We were definitely not on our own now. I was still a student and I knew that jobs like this thankfully don't happen every day. But they do happen and I needed to learn all I could, so that if a similar incident came along when I was registered and qualified, I could work from what I had learned. I put on my helmet and high visibility coat and was there waiting to get on the tracks with other members of staff. Once the power was off, I climbed down and we walked along the train tracks until we reached the point where his body was lying. I remember his face clearly: his grey complexion and lifeless eyes. His eyes were still open and staring up at the sky. I wished someone would close them but I didn't have the courage to do it myself.

I thought he would have looked far more peaceful, instead of having the horrendous expression that was on his face. I worked together with the other members of various teams to officially confirm his death. I remember thinking that all the checks to confirm death had a touch of 'overkill' (an inappropriate term, I know). The man's torso was barely attached to his lower limbs. There was just a bit of fatty muscle tissue and skin here and there holding it all together. His entire blood volume was sloshing around in his stomach for Christ sake, so why we needed to prod and pull this poor man around more to definitively say he was dead was beyond me. But these are the things we must do.

After speaking to the train driver and hearing information relayed from the CCTV it appeared that this gentleman intentionally ended his own life by climbing down onto the tracks as the train approached and lying across the rails.

He had a picture of a woman and two kids in his wallet.

19

Watch Her Resp's As She Could Stop Breathing

One of the first seizures I saw was in a 10-year-old girl. The scary part is that if the Mum had not told me she was having a seizure I would probably never have guessed. Of course, my mentor would have spotted the signs, but not me. This little girl was lying in her urine-soaked bed, not moving at all. Now, usually you would expect people having a convulsion, or fitting, (whatever term you are familiar with) to be shaking in their arms and legs. But not all seizures present this way. You can have focal seizures, which just involves one part of the body, or you can have absence seizures, where no parts move. You can mostly identify these kinds of seizures from the patient's eyes. As a qualified paramedic, I have had one child go into an absent seizure in my care and I noticed it from observing the eyes. They were twitching back and forth and wouldn't fix onto any stimulus you put in front of them.

With this 10-year-old girl in her bed, we already knew she was in an absent seizure. Her Mum explained that it was normal for her to have them, but she wasn't coming out of this one. Her normal one lasted about five minutes but this one was coming up to ten minutes. She had had her buccal Midazolam medication which is meant to help relax the muscles and stop the seizure. It had been ineffective.

One of the key things to remember when someone is having a seizure is that the person can quickly become starved of oxygen. It is often difficult to breathe when having a seizure so the sufferer can become blue or pale. So, we quickly placed high flow oxygen onto her via a high flow mask. This quickly corrected her low oxygen levels. The next step was to get her out of the small, cluttered bedroom and into a space where we had more room to work.

We decided to take her straight out to the ambulance so we could administer diazepam. I had never given diazepam at this point and was shown how to by another medic on the scene. As the girl was too difficult to cannulate the medicine had to be given via the rectum. We were coming up to nearly 20 minutes of continuous fitting; after a few minutes of giving the rectal diazepam we soon realised that the medication wasn't working and she needed to be blued into the nearest hospital. As we made our way to the hospital the paramedic sitting with me in the back said 'Watch her resp's – she could stop breathing... you will need to bag her if she does.' I looked at the medic in horror and thought: *Why on earth would she stop breathing?* Now I have come to know better and never assume anything when it comes to children. Take every precaution and cover every base.

Thankfully she kept her own respiratory rate quite nicely, but once we were in hospital it did start to decline again and she was intubated and sedated to try and regain control over her body. The Mum did amazingly – she was so brave and understanding throughout. I don't know if I would be able to be that calm if my child was that poorly. Despite all the hospital's efforts she was still convulsing when it was time for us to leave the hospital.

I had a mixed bag of jobs in my last year as a student: from heart attacks, strokes, cardiac arrests, children having seizures, and drunks, to assaults. I had an amazing mentor who made me feel confident in my decisions and my practice – but I still had so much to learn. There were so many experiences I still needed to see and feel while having the support of a mentor by my side. One time, we went to a cardiac arrest of an elderly lady who had died suddenly at home with her husband while watching telly. Her husband had called an ambulance and the call taker had instructed him how to do CPR. So, when we arrived on the scene, he was performing CPR on his wife, in floods of tears.

We did everything we could for this lady, but sadly she had passed away. The husband grabbed my hand at the end and asked me if he had done it right and whether this was all his fault. The strength it took for me to hold back tears and reassure him that he had done an amazing job but that unfortunately it had just been her time to go, was unbelievable.

This man had just lost his wife and we were there as professionals: I couldn't start tearing up and sobbing in his house! I haven't experienced such loss in my life and I'm lucky for that, so it's hard to find the right words sometimes. I don't always know what to say to a patient or family members when it's all going wrong, and I worry that I might not ever get better at this. You do, sadly. But at the time I was worried that I would arrive in the big bad world with my shiny new paramedic status and completely fuck it up.

IV

Graduation and Qualification

20

Love, Certificates & Congratulations

We made it to graduation and qualification. It wouldn't be right to talk about this stage of my life without talking about the man in my life, who was with me throughout this stage. We met at the end of third year, right in the middle of all my exams. I messed him around a few times, actually once deciding to study instead of going on a date, a decision that I am proud of myself for making. But thank God – he gave me another chance.

When we finally got around to that first date, I can say that by the time I drank my first glass of wine I knew I had met the man I was going to marry. I was completely head over heels in love and still am to this day. Thankfully my feelings were reciprocated and we moved in together just two months after our first date.

We now have a dog and are well on our way to buying our first home! Coming home to him every night, no matter how hard the shift was, makes the whole day worthwhile. He brightens my mood even if I'm in the darkest place and I could never be without this man. God bless you for putting up with me and my crazy work schedule. I love you.

Well, that time had come, graduation day. The big bad world and all that crap. I felt an enormous amount of pride when I was collecting my certificate: BSc Honours degree in Paramedic Science. My family and boyfriend were in the crowd and I really felt like I had finally achieved something they were proud of!

We continued the day with prosecco and a fancy meal. It was beautiful and I definitely fell asleep that night with a smile on my face and not a worry in the world. During the build up to graduation I had spent my time applying for jobs. I had had a couple of part-time jobs to get me through University but I really wanted to jump straight from university to work. Thankfully this is what happened.

I applied for the London Ambulance Service (LAS) and got accepted for an interview! After doing three years training on the road with them you would think you'd at least get an interview but this wasn't automatically the case. You had to apply just like everyone else, and pretty much write an essay telling them why you should even be considered for an interview.

I went to the interview with a friend as she had also applied for the London Ambulance Service and we nervously made our way to London. I was called up to have my interview. In front of me were three members of staff, and blimey, did they look intimidating! One member of the panel was in smart office attire and the other two in full LAS uniform, and they seemed like they were high up the professional ladder. They asked me why I wanted to work for the LAS, and what LAS's values are; what my idea of patient care was; and what my idea of dignity and respect was: those kinds of things. I don't know why, but I have always been good at those kinds of interviews. Bullshit with conviction, they say! But on a serious note, I honestly do like that style of questioning because, as long as you don't say something ridiculous, it is just your own opinion. They just want to know if you share the same opinions as they do.

The second part of the interview was a test on clinical knowledge and this part terrified me. I had professional managing paramedics asking me clinical questions that I had to get bang on, otherwise I would not only look stupid but incompetent. I answered the first two questions confidently and professionally and maybe they thought I did a little too well because one of the interviewers decided to ask me a 'tricky' question and I completely choked. I had no idea what the answer was – or even what he was talking about! I must have impressed them earlier on though, because I was offered a job and I know that some people were turned down for messing up on the clinical questions. I was completely ecstatic after receiving my congratulations phone call! Well, I say congratulations – it was quite an anti-climax because the person on the other end of the phone was clearly having a bad day!

'Hello is this *****?'

'Hi, yes, speaking...' By this point, I knew it was a London number calling so I'm sweating and frozen in place.

'Hello, it's Carol from recruitment at London Ambulance Service, I'm glad to say you have been accepted and we would like to offer you a job with us.' Good old Carol told me this amazing news in the most monotone voice you can imagine!

'Oh, wow, that's amazing thank you!'

'Yes, well done.' (It still sounds like she is telling me about paint drying) 'When are you able to start?'

'Erm, I'm not too sure, as soon as possible I guess!'

'Great I'll send over the details, thanks.' That was pretty much it for my congratulations! But, hey, Carol may have been miserable – but I was over the moon! I ran to my friend and told her the news. However, she still hadn't found out about her application, so we were both anxious to see if she also got the job! (She did receive a congratulations call a few hours later from a much happier lady!)

I started a few months later which involved five weeks in a classroom and four weeks training for my blue light driving exam. I passed it all. I then went on to do ten weeks training on the road – this stage was called OPC (Operational Placement Centre). I had a mentor who was a band 6 medic, and also on the truck was another NQP1 (Newly Qualified Paramedic) training with me. This is like your buffer period, so you can go out as a registered paramedic and perform the skills you have trained for, but you have a bit of back up to support you.

This job is funny. You can have weeks of run-of-the-mill jobs, like back pain, severe headaches, abdominal pain, and even down to common colds. Then all of a sudden you will have a triple shooting and you're the only crew on the scene with armed police shouting at you to tell them what to do... (Yes, this happened to me, more on that later).

The ten weeks flew by, and this helped as I had a fantastic mentor, my confidence was growing and I really felt like I was getting somewhere and achieving my goals. I found my patient assessments were flowing, my treatment plans were on point and everything was dandy in the world. I had so many new exciting things making life amazing and challenging, and I loved it. Of course, I was still sheltered in the bubble of always having someone around me with my patients. Even when I was treating someone in the back, I would have the other NQP1 with me for the tricky jobs. There was a constant team there to bounce ideas off and ask: 'What do you think about this treatment?'; 'Shall we try this?'; 'You know, it could be this that's causing that!' So, by the time I left OPC, I felt great, but I also knew that these exciting, confident times were short-lived and I was about to be really challenged. And if I'm honest I was dreading it!

21

Are You Kidding Me!

My first day officially on relief had begun, I was crewed up with another paramedic and it was just me and him on the road. This was the first time ever in my career that it had been just me and another crewmate in the truck. I introduced myself and felt the need to inform him pretty quickly that this was my first day out on relief. He was sweet about it; in a perfect world he would have offered to attend all shift and let me settle in, but realistically that wasn't going to happen because I needed to man the hell up and just throw myself into it.

All the while I was praying that it would be an easy day. The first half of the shift was nice and chilled and my crewmate attended for it; I was driving as I legally could now! We got to the change over time of the shift and it was my turn to jump into the attendant's seat. I gathered my bits together and prepared myself for the job that was about to come in. Before we green up (become available for a job), we radio through to our sector and ask for a job back in area, in the hope of finishing our shift in our local area. The problem is you can be called to areas all around London and that will only make you finish late.

'Hello sector, we're coming up to the end of our shift – you got anything back in area to see us off?'

'Hey, yep, I do, I'll ping it to you now if you go green, apologise.'

Why is he saying 'apologise'? I wondered.

My crewmate looked at me in disbelief at what had come through the screen.

'Fucks sake, why is this a CAT 2?' He started up the truck and switched on the lights, speeding through the traffic. I look at the screen and panicked at the sight of 'Peri-Arrest'. That's all that was given but it was enough for me. My first fully unsupervised job as a paramedic and I am the attending paramedic to an elderly man who is actively dying. That sounds a bit silly, but that is exactly what 'peri-arrest' means. He was about to arrest and whatever the reason was, he was going to die soon if we didn't get there fast and try to save his life.

I like to run things through in my head – but out loud – this might not be everyone's cup of tea but that's how I feel. I organise my thoughts, and also the person I am working with then knows what my thought process is, and they can then add something that I may have missed out. My first words after reading the job were rather unprofessional but what can you say? I'm only human.

'Are you fucking kidding me! Fuck, OK, we will take in full resus kit and the bed, correct any A & B problems (airway & breathing) and as soon as we can, we run.' (take to hospital). The reason I don't say C (circulation) at this point is because, unless his blood pressure is in his boots and dropping, or he has lost a limb, most corrections for circulation can be time-consuming or get out of our control. Every job is different and when you see a patient you kind of have an idea of what things to check, and what things can wait till you have a little more time to investigate. We arrived at the care home and struggled to find anyone to let us in. Then, once we were in, no one seemed to know where we were going. You would be surprised how many times an organisation will call for an ambulance but actually no one knows where the patient is! We were directed to the common room and I no longer needed the assistance of the care worker as I had seen my patient. A nurse was bent over a frail elderly gentleman in an armchair performing a jaw thrust with high flow oxygen on. The gentleman looked grey and was moaning and clawing at the nurse, in hypoxic agitation. I got to the nurse with my bags and started connecting equipment, then asked: 'Hey what's happened?'

'I came in to do his meds and saw him slumped over, barely breathing. He looked grey so I got the oxygen on and his sats were showing at 60% on room air. I haven't been able to do much else as he has been fighting the mask...'

'No, that's great,' I looked at the monitor and saw his oxygen was about 81% on 15L of oxygen. That was not great at all.

'Let's get the pads on and move him on to our oxygen.' I have a quick listen to his chest and it was unbelievably crackly at the top of the lobes and completely silent at the bottom. I was thinking at this point he had pneumonia or some kind of chest infection. We quickly moved him on the bed by grabbing any part of his body that we could and lifting in one swift heave. His heart rate was all over the place and the rhythm was something out of my scope of practice. His heart was beating, but not very well at all. Once on the trolley bed with a better view we could see he had good chest rise and fall, but was breathing very erratically. We grabbed all the bags and headed to the truck; sometimes people just need to be in hospital – we could 'stay and play' all we wanted but it just wouldn't make a difference. I called out to the group of carers standing staring (one of whom was drinking TEA!): 'Have you got his personal details for us to take?!'

'Erm... yeah, do you want them?'

'YES, quickly please, we really aren't going to be here long, also does he have a DNR? If so, can you please bring it as that's very important.' If you don't know, a DNR means 'Do Not Resuscitate'. This is a certificate that declares the decision the patient or the family have made, which means if they are to die, we are not to perform any ventilations or attempts to bring that person back to life. Palliative care patients usually have this in place, so they are to be kept comfortable until they pass unless there are any reversible causes: otherwise, they are essentially left to die in peace.

'Yeah, I think he does have one of those.'

'OK well it's really important we see it – we can't go off your word unfortunately.' All DNR must be witnessed by the crew or doctors, you can't just be told by family or friends that he didn't want to be resuscitated. It has to be an official document signed by a doctor. I really want to see this certificate because something tells me this gentleman isn't going to survive and the last thing I want to do is start jumping on his chest and pumping him full of drugs if all he wanted was to die in peace.

Minutes had passed and we were in the truck: there were no details and no certificate. One of the ladies who worked at the care home came out to say they couldn't find his file. So, we decided to leave without them as we had no choice. His oxygen levels were fluctuating and he was becoming more aggressive.

My crewmate jumped in the front of the truck and put through the blue call, I continued the jaw thrust to try and open up his airway while looking at his oxygen levels and his breathing. He was breathing extremely quickly and his CO_2 levels were all over the place. I remember standing with this man's head in my hands, forcing his jaw open, with a series of thoughts running through my head. They went kind of like this:

Fuck, what am I doing?

Is this right?

What button do I press if he died and I need to shock him?

Are the pads plugged in?

Shit, I didn't get the bag valve mask out in case I need to breathe for him.

Shit, I should have done a 12-lead ECG on him.

I can't move my hands.

Should I put in an airway? Will he tolerate an airway? Probably not.

Fuck, what's that noise coming from the machine, why is that alarm going off?

Is he breathing?

Damn it, I should have put a cannula in as well, was there time?

Fuck what is that coming out of his mouth?!

That would be vomit, which was now coming out of the airway, I was trying so hard to keep it clear, so with one hand holding the oxygen mask over his mouth, the other grabbed the suction kit, which of course I hadn't set up before we left the scene: so this was also being assembled. I started to suction the phlegm, vomit and spit coming out of his mouth and noticed an increase in his oxygen levels! Oh shit, it's working, I looked at the oxygen levels that were now sitting at 90% and I was beaming.

That doesn't last long unfortunately, and they started to drop quickly again so I tried a new tactic to keep him alive until we got to the hospital. One hand held the mask down as he was still trying to claw my hands and my face, while the other was suctioning his airway to keep it clear.

We FINALLY got to the hospital, which seemed like far too long, and the back of the truck looked like a bomb had gone off: there was kit everywhere and in the middle was me, red-faced, sweating, and completely terrified (on the inside). I still don't know if what I did was right or wrong because, to be honest, the whole thing happened in a blur and I was in the back on my own for what must have been about 10 minutes. But for those 10 minutes I felt completely alone. My crewmate was a shout away but the fear and stress I felt in those ten minutes: *Please God keep this man alive a little longer, just a little longer* is beyond words. MY FIRST PATIENT.

I couldn't make it up if I tried. I remember sitting in the truck after that job in a state of shock thinking to myself: *Oh damn, I'm so not ready for this.*

I wasn't organised enough; I didn't think ahead enough. I had no idea what I was doing. I needed to seriously up my game if I was going to be able to make this a career, and for the first time in four years I wondered if this was the job for me.

I drove home that night and cried pretty much all the way home. I didn't want to go back to work because I didn't under any circumstances want to feel that way again. That gut-wrenching fear that it's all going wrong and someone's life is in your hands. The responsibility is enormous and I only really appreciated that on the drive home after that day.

Next day I woke up, jumped in the shower, got dressed, and drove back into work. *Today will be a better day,* I thought.

Six Months Later

OK, don't worry. I'm not about to say that I quit work and never went back after that day because that isn't true and this book would be pretty pointless if it was. I was however still suffering with anxiety driving into work. My hands felt sweaty and my heart would pound when I saw the ambulance station. But what else could I do but keep turning up every day? It wasn't going to get better unless I kept going. I sometimes thought about backing out, but the thought would be quickly squashed by me thinking: *Don't you dare!*

I was working with people that I could confide in and open up to about my worries and fears, and I got the impression that it was pretty normal to feel the way I did, and that it never really goes away! Great.

I can say with some certainty that I will always have this anxiety in this job. I now realise that it is not a bad thing either: if you don't have that fear and pit of worry then you may become complacent and cocky, which is one of the worst attitudes to bring into healthcare.

Jobs can surprise you at any turn, you need to be alert and ready to change treatment and pace at any point. I have become more organised and proactive but there is always room to learn and improve. Jobs along the way have trained me to better myself as a paramedic. In my opinion, no amount of classroom practice and online training can fully get you there. Unfortunately, my degree taught me *half* my knowledge and I have learned the other half from my mistakes or experiences. Or shall I say near-mistakes. Because we don't make mistakes… right?

22

Just Breathe Bridget

Never in my wildest dreams did I think I would swear at a patient but God, I swore at Bridget. Thankfully she was this little Irish lady and she cracked up at me telling her to shut up. It still didn't help her breathing though. We were called to Bridget on a sunny Sunday: they are a rare occurrence in the UK, so I was lapping up the sun whenever I could. The job came down as an asthma attack. This was pretty common at that point due to the erratic weather we were having – one minute cold, the next baking hot.

I was attending and I have this thing where I MUST put on gloves before I get to the patient. I don't want to be caught out one day delivering a baby or grabbing a vomit-covered t-shirt without gloves on, so before I even get out of the truck, the gloves are on. My crewmate for this particular job had seen the patient coming out of the house and started walking towards her before I was out of the truck. I saw the pair of them heading to the truck with her suitcase in hand. My thoughts were: *Ah bless, she has packed a bag ready to go to hospital.* I walked to the far side of the truck and opened the door ready for them to jump in, taking it for granted that if she was walking out to us with her bags packed, then she couldn't be that bad.

Well, they made it to the door, but she looked grey and was clearly using every muscle she could to breathe – each breath looked like she was sucking in as hard as she possibly could to puff the smallest amount of air back out. The wheeze was so audible – I could hear it as they turned the corner of the truck.

Oh shit, I thought, *she is not OK.* I grabbed her by the scruff of her dressing gown and told my crewmate to give her a bump up. I pulled and he pushed and up she came. She fell slumped onto the chair. All the while she was rambling on: 'So… rry I …. cal … led … you … gu..ys… I'm… struggling… to… bre… athe … this… bloo… dy… asth… ma.'

'Bridget, don't worry about it, just focus on your breathing for now, and we will sort you out.' I put the stats probe on her finger and it gave me a reading of 61%. Not good at all. 'Can you get a neb sorted please mate?' I asked my crewmate as I listened to her chest. 'Ye…ah…its…the….wea…ther….cha… nge'

'Bridget, it's fine, we can talk about that in a minute. I really just want you to breathe that nebuliser in for a few minutes and get your lungs sounding a bit better.'

'OK… dear… it's… ju… st… I… tri… ed… my… pu… mps…'

'Bridget, it's fine, we will sort you out, it sounds like a nasty asthma attack: do you also have COPD? Just nod to me, yes or no.'

'Yes… de… ar… I… ha… ve… had… C…O… P…D'

'BRIDGET! No talking please – your oxygen levels are low… just breathe that salbutamol in. Is it helping at all… just nod for me…'

'Yes… this… stuffs… gre… at…' However, she was still as grey as my Grandad's facial hair, and her oxygen levels were… shit, to put it bluntly.

'Bridget, shut up and breathe!' I said, half laughing and half exasperated. Thankfully, Bridget just started cracking up laughing, much to my appreciation, and thankfully she showed she had listened by placing one finger over her mouth to symbolise silence. I knew deep down she would enjoy the humour from her bubbly personality despite her unwell state.

'Thank you, right, let's have a listen to that chest.' It was sounding slightly better, but not by much, and her oxygen levels weren't holding up well. We decided to blue her in to hospital for acute exacerbation of asthma and COPD. Now, this job was also a learning curve for me – firstly because you should not swear at patients, even if in jest. So, it wasn't very professional on my part. Secondly, I spent so much time trying to stop her talking, but also to be kind enough to listen to her chat away as she clearly hadn't seen someone to talk to in a few weeks, that I completely forgot to treat what we were actually there to treat. I left her on 6L of oxygen, trying not to flood her with oxygen due to her COPD. She really could have done with some drugs such as ipratropium bromide to help open up her airways and she probably wouldn't have struggled as much as she did on the way to hospital – but for some reason I didn't. I got distracted.

When we arrived at the hospital, she was alive and relatively well, but she was still fighting for breath and chewing the ear off the nurses who were taking over. The doctor asked how much atrovent (drug brand name) she had had. I froze and remembered I hadn't given it to her. Why? I don't bloody know. It wasn't a mistake that cost her her life, but I still couldn't wrap my head around why I had become so side-tracked by Bridget chatting away that I had forgotten to treat her!

Distractions are part of the job; they come in various different forms on a daily basis, and the hard part is separating what's important from what is not. I wouldn't say I am a perfectionist, but I have found in this job that little things can bother me for days. Like: *Why didn't I ask that question? Why didn't I try that? Or: I should have written that paperwork a lot neater!*

I like to think it is because I am passionate about what I do, but it could just be that I'm secretly terrified for the day something goes wrong.

23

Wait You Can't Leave Me

Unfortunately, traumas such as stabbings and shootings are on the rise in London. People are attacked and then in retaliation the attackers are themselves attacked and it just goes on and on. You may have seen the anti-knife campaign in and around London in bus stops and on billboards aimed at raising awareness. Basically – just stop bloody stabbing each other!

I went to a job not too long ago for a 10-year-old boy who had fallen on a climbing frame in the park across from his block of flats. He was back in the flat by the time I had arrived, but you could see the entrance to the park from the window and something else caught my eye more – the blue and white tape closing off part of the estate. 'What happened here?' I asked. 'Oh there was a stabbing last night, it was on the news… did you not hear about it?'

'No, I must have missed it.' If I'm honest, I don't watch the news, I hear enough shit and see some horrible stuff in my day-to-day job, so to be watching it when I get home is a 'no' from me. Home is my bubble. News doesn't make the cut in my bubble. The thought crossed my mind that even though there had been a stabbing in the same street the night before, there was still a group of kids ranging from 8-13 years old playing in the park on the same street the next evening! But I guess it is so normal for these families that life just carries on. The sight of a crime scene outside your window is sadly normal, and there's nothing that can be done about it, so you just carry on with your day and act as if it isn't there.

I had only been to one shooting in my career prior to the job I'm about to describe, and that had been as a student. Thankfully the young girl I mentioned earlier in this book had been completely fine, so no real clinical interventions were needed, but it was still baffling that this stuff happened in England.

My first proper shooting was very different. I was crewed up with another paramedic that had been a student at the time. In a weird way it felt like we were both students, and it was a great comfort to me when she asked questions and I actually knew the answers and could help her out.

During a night shift we were sitting at the station waiting for a job. It's not often that it happens where we are green and waiting with a cup of tea for the next job to come in. Usually, it's all just *go go go*. But for a change we had ten minutes to sit and scroll through our phones with a lovely hot cup of tea and a few bickies. The job came in as CAT1. Of course!

As you can imagine, when you receive a job through the hand-held radio you don't get full details. It will mostly say the category of the job, the age and gender of the patient, and maybe you might get a little bit of an idea of what the job is about, or it will just be an address. For this job we could just see a street name. We gathered our bits and rushed to the truck to get back out onto the road. Once we all climbed back into our seats, with me in the driver's seat, we saw the update come down the screen of what the job actually was. This is roughly what we saw on the screen:

Age UK Gender UK NO. OF PT: 3 Breathing Y Conscious N Shooting. Shooter whereabouts unknown. 3 patients identified.

So, I'll break this down: UK means unknown, the number of patients so far is three! Y means yes and N would mean no. So, at the moment they are breathing but one or all three aren't conscious. I started driving, and it was probably some of my best driving on blue lights because I was getting the truck through spaces that I probably wouldn't try my Mini in. As I bombed it down the motorway, I could hear the police hot on my tail. For shootings or stabbings, police must be on the scene first to make sure the area is safe: we will wait at a rendezvous area to be told to come in when it is safe to do so. A second later, two large blacked-out BMWs shot past on blue lights: that was armed police and thankfully they were going to get there before us!

We weren't far away, and we ran through what was going to happen when we got there as a team. 'Right, we make sure it is safe to go to the patient because by the sounds of it they don't have the shooter, we stop the bleeding, try and find all the sources, high flow oxygen and get them on the bed and go as soon as possible. Lines in on the road if we have time or in the truck when more back up comes. Sounds good?' 'Sounds good.'

I was praying they have more trucks or cars available at this point because we were at the street just before where the shooting was said to have taken place, and the police weren't anywhere to be seen. I wasn't sure how, as they had passed us, but we were here first.

I looked around frantically to see if I had made a wrong turn somewhere or if we were on the right street. 'PLEASE, THIS WAY THEY'RE OVER HERE!'A young guy was shouting and waving at me from the side of the truck. 'Fuck, the patient's there!' I looked out of the front window and saw a group of lads by a male lying in the middle of the road behind some cars. The black BMW pulled up to the side of us in the same instant and a sigh of relief came over me.

We jumped out and grabbed the necessary kit then started making our way over to the patient. I take my hat off to the police. When it comes to trauma jobs, they are QUICK at stopping the bleeding and assessing a patient. There's no messing around. By the time we had got out of the truck, got our bags and reached the patient, his clothes had been cut off and there was a tourniquet and bandage on his left leg stopping the bleeding. 'We have stopped the bleeding; I think it is just one entry and exit point in the upper left thigh.'

'Amazing guys, thank you.' My crewmate tapped me on the shoulder and grabbed the medic bag: 'There are two more over here. I'll go triage them; you treat this guy.'

'Wait, what?!' I looked over in a panic as he left me with at least five police officers and a patient bleeding out from his leg. I thought to myself: *Wait, you can't leave me I'm only a student.* And then the realisation came pretty quickly: *Oh wait, damn, I'm not a student any more, I've actually got to run this.*

'What do you need us to do?' The officer shouted at me and I had a surreal moment looking at the group of butch, intimidating police officers waiting for a command from me. I had armed police telling me the area was secure for now and asking if I needed any help transporting the patient or needed any kit.

WHAT THE HELL IS GOING ON! It felt like a long minute of me staring at them and staring at the patient. It was probably only about seven seconds, but that drags when you don't have a bloody clue what to say or what to do! Then it was almost like a switch went off in my head. *Grow the hell up,* I said to myself *and do your job.*

'Right Jessie, go get the trolley bed and board from the truck.' My student ran off.

'Do you know how to set the oxygen up?' A police officer nodded yes to my question.

'Great, you do that please, and on 15L.' I checked his body once more for any other sources of bleeding but it did seem to be just the one. Then I checked his radial to see how his blood pressure was holding up – it was weak but I could feel it. If someone's radial pulse is too weak to feel, that usually means their blood pressure has taken a severe drop. The young male was crying out in pain, which is also a good sign: the noisier the better, I say. My crewmate came back to see me and my team working away on this patient and I felt a sense of pride: I had this job under control, somehow!

'OK, boards on either side, we can move him to the bed, once clipped together each grab a corner and lift when I say, lift.' My crewmate told me the other two patients were stable and there was another medic on the scene treating them. We lifted the patient and started getting him to the truck, and as we did, HEMS. Remember I told you before, they are like the grown-ups of trauma: well praise Jesus they were here. I give them a brief handover as to what had happened – by the sounds of it, it had been a drive-by shooting in which the shooter had hit them all in the legs. Thankfully no one was critical by the time we were transporting them to hospital. And no other bystanders or emergency services had been injured. Apparently, the shooter had driven past on a moped and opened fire on a group of men standing by the side of the road. What their reason for this was, I'll never know but to have that much hate in you to not care who or what you hit with a firearm still baffles me. To be so careless with life: it has become the sad world we live in.

We continued to treat this gentleman all the way to a major trauma centre in London, with an armed escort all the way there and into the hospital. There is something about the armed police guys and women – they look bloody terrifying. It's probably the array of guns they have strapped to them, but I found myself talking to this officer like a silly school girl talking to their headmaster: 'Thank you for all your help guys, you did great.'

Bloody hell, get me out of here before I say something stupid like 'nice guns'.

24

What's Wrong With Her Heart

A few chapters back, I spoke about my fear of paediatric jobs. Well, this incident is one of the reasons for that fear. Before I became registered, I used to have the thought process: *Ah, I like children, I don't mind the paediatric jobs.* How naive I was when I had no responsibilities! I do now, and this young girl was my first big sick paediatric job that I attended. In the back of the ambulance, with her being blue lighted to hospital, the whole time I was praying: *Please God, don't die.*

This is probably not a new piece of information to most people, but children have a tendency to be coping very well with their illness, whatever it may be, and then their bodies just give up: they decline incredibly quickly and it's important to realise when or if they are going to reach that threshold. Not every child with a chest infection is going to need an ambulance or hospital admission, but it's always good to know the warning signs for when a child is big sick. If you have young children, research your sepsis markers for the age of your child. Listen on YouTube to hear what cough sounds aren't simply just a cough. Know every medication your child is on and all the details of any medical conditions your child has.

Many mothers and fathers reading this may be thinking, what a silly statement that is to make, because of course they do all that. However, you will be surprised at how many times I ask 'What's this medication for?' and the answer is 'Oh, I think it's for this?' Small things can catch you out, like the side effects of medication. Please, please read about the side effects before giving your child medication, so you are aware of what could happen! My brother fell victim to this when his child was rushed to hospital with red flag sepsis: its source was a chest infection. He noticed his son had a cough and high temperature and was treating it with Calpol, but it wasn't until he took his son's shirt off and someone else noticed that his breathing looked odd that he decided enough was enough and took him to hospital.

His son was struggling to breathe so much that his oxygen levels were dangerously low and he was doing something called intercostal recession breathing. This is where you are using all your muscles to breathe effectively, and trying to do this so hard that it is actually causing the skin and muscle in between the ribs to suck in with every breath. He told me: 'He was fine, running around playing, and then all of a sudden he lay down on the floor and I just thought he had become over tired from playing.' It was actually that my nephew's infection had really caught up with him and his body couldn't handle the work anymore.

The case I want to describe is a three-year-old young girl I went to. She wasn't suffering from a chest infection like her mother had initially thought. So, I'll start from the beginning.

We were called to her because she was struggling to breathe and her hands were turning blue. Obviously, straight off the bat this doesn't sound like a good job, and I was already incredibly nervous about the situation. I always get my mini book out (otherwise known as JRCALC, which is basically a quick-look guide to drugs we carry and triage tools) and write down some details, such as normal heart rate, respiratory rate, blood pressure and possible drug dosages for someone of her age. As they vary so much in children you don't want to be thinking a respiratory rate of 14 is OK for a three-year-old when actually it should be more for people in their 20s.

Adult vital signs are completely different from children and that should never be forgotten. Also, if a child is indeed big sick, the last thing you want to be doing is rummaging through a book to find the correct figures. Get this all prepared before arriving. Always cross-checking everything is key, as having a basic idea when you walk into a job is extremely helpful. So, we arrived at the flat for this young girl and a neighbour flagged us down at the front door: she seemed smiley and friendly. This seemed to lessen the sense of urgency. Of course, we still proceeded expecting the worst but if someone is standing there smiling and laughing about how many flights of stairs we have just climbed, then really how ill can the child be? We walk in and I ask where the patient is: 'Oh she is in the living room,' the woman said.

'Lovely, thank you, are you Mum?' I always call the parents 'Mum' and 'Dad' when around paediatric patients, I feel like it may put the child more at ease than calling them by the proper names.

'No, she is in the living room, I'm her neighbour.'

'Ah OK, no worries,' As I walked through the door, I saw a

young girl lying on the sofa in a ball. Her knees were to her chest and her face pressed against the sofa. She raised her head to look at who had walked in and instantly cried at seeing us. I would say she was struggling to breathe because she was probably breathing at a rate of 45-50 breaths a minute and she was sweating buckets. It was actually quite horrific to see.

'What happened?' The Mum unfortunately spoke very little English so the neighbour intervened to answer.

'She has had a fever, we think since this morning, and she has been breathing fast like this since then.'

'She has been like this all day!' We are at roughly 3pm at this point. I tried to approach the young girl without scaring her, using the friendliest calmest voice I could, as she was quite clearly terrified and very distressed. My crewmate, without scaring the child too much, managed to get a temperature from the patient, which came back normal. This puzzled me: at first my diagnosis was a bad chest infection which had progressed to her becoming septic. Usually, a fever is a key indicator. This is not always the case as some infections or diagnoses can fluctuate with fever. But something wasn't adding up.

'We need to get some layers off her, as she is sweating like mad.' I leaned over to my crewmate and together we were able to get her t-shirt off. I wanted to listen to her breathing to see if she needed a nebuliser. I had already decided that we were not going to hang around on this job as this little girl needed to be seen by a doctor quickly but I also wanted to make sure there was nothing I could do treatment-wise at that moment that would make her feel better.

'Has she been having Calpol?'

'Yes, she had some about an hour ago,' said the neighbour, after translating from the mother. The layers of clothing were finally off and now I was presented with a massive scar in the middle of her chest.

'What is this?! Has she had open heart surgery?' Bearing in mind one of my first questions is always whether there is any previous medical conditions, to which the mother had answered no.

'Oh, she said she had had heart surgery,' said the neighbour.

'Yes, I can see that, but what was it for?'

'Erm... she does not know.' I looked at my crewmate in concern and horror that this was probably a lot more complicated than an infection.

'Right, we have to go, we need to connect her to a machine downstairs called an ECG. It will do a reading of her heart. Can you get your bits like keys, wallet and phone and let's go,' I scooped up the little girl in my arms: she was now a lot quieter and seemed to be cuddling me. The Mum started packing the baby bag which was clearly not for the three-year-old. She also had a three-week-old newborn lying in the living room sleeping.

'You really shouldn't be taking a newborn to A&E. We will be going to resus which is in the main A&E and your baby could become very ill in such an infectious place as a hospital.'

The neighbour explained that no one was there to look after the baby. After I questioned her, she explained she couldn't watch the baby as she didn't like to because the baby cried too much.

'No, I'm sorry... do you have milk all set up in the fridge?' The mother and neighbour nod to my question.

'Great, we need to go now, so can you watch the baby until Dad comes home and Mum, we need to go now. We are going to walk her down, please be quick.' The neighbour looked pissed off but there was a reason for my bluntness. Actually a few. One was that this child was extremely sick: anyone could see that so why they had let her sit like this ALL day was beyond me. The second was annoyance that she had complained about looking after a sleeping newborn because they cry, regardless of the fact that it allowed Mum to come with us to the hospital on her own. Thirdly, the ambulance is not equipped to take two young children safely. The patient is going to need the bed. The idea of strapping a car seat into the seats in the ambulance on a blue call sends shivers down my spine and my focus needs to be on the three-year-old, so I can't be worrying about a car seat and whether it is stable enough to transport.

So, yes, the pair unfortunately experienced me at my snappy 'Don't take the piss' stage. This poor child wasn't just unwell, she was big sick, hospitalisation sick, and how these ladies couldn't see that was beyond me.

When we arrived, the little girl was pale white, sweating and her arms and legs were blue. She was seriously deprived of oxygen. We made it to the ambulance, attached the young girl to equipment and started to create a picture of what was really going on with her, before the mother had even left the house. From doing the ECG we learned she was in fact suffering with something called supraventricular tachycardia, otherwise known as SVT. This is where the heart is beating far too fast. Her young heart rate was sitting at 260 bpm. We had no idea how long it had been this way but from the look of her it had been a while. During our journey downstairs she had settled enough in my arms for me to put oxygen on her in the hope that it would help her. Now I knew that she definitely needed the oxygen.

She was still incredibly blue in her hands and feet but I really wasn't surprised at this point. Another problem with paediatric jobs is that our sats probes, which tell us a person's oxygen levels, don't fit little children and it's very difficult to get an accurate reading. But at this point I really didn't need to use it to see that this child needed oxygen. The Mum finally got on the back of the truck and my crewmate jumped in the front to begin the blue light drive to the nearest hospital.

Do you remember earlier that I said I never wanted to be caught off guard again with a patient? Well for her, I had everything ready. I had the defibrillator machine placed at the end of the bed with the pads attached to her, in case her heart gave out (which was quite a high probability at that point). I also had a bag valve mask next to her in case I needed to manually ventilate her during transit.

I just sat on the bed with her and prayed. I am not a religious woman but sometimes it just feels like it helps. Unfortunately, for a child in SVT there really isn't anything we ambulance staff can do There could be things we could try with adults, but not with children. The little girl started to seem vacant with me during the journey and my heart began to sink. I was trying desperately to get her to interact with me to make sure she was still there, and that her body hadn't given out from the exhaustion.

Was she becoming so hypoxic that her brain wasn't being perfused properly? I looked over to Mum to try and explain to her what was going on and what we were trying to do for her: due to the language barrier I tried my best, but struggled. She spent much of the time on her phone texting and calling people, I imagine to tell loved ones to what was happening.

'You can hold her hand if you want,' the mum looked at me and then her child and moved forward to hold her hand in reassurance.

When we arrived at the hospital, her heart rate was at 270. Like any muscle, if you use it too much, it will become tired and could just stop working. This was my fear, and by the time we had pulled up I had grabbed a portable oxygen cylinder and disconnected the patient from the machines. Correct procedure would have been to take her in on the bed, but I really felt we didn't have time so I grabbed her and ran her into resus. It must have looked ridiculous, me carrying a child in my arms with an oxygen cylinder in one hand and defibrillator pads dangling around this young girl's legs, but I knew I needed some help and the quicker she was in with the doctors the better.

The doctors and nurses quickly recognised my panicked face and shot into action to hear what was going on and start treatment. The hustle and bustle of a seriously ill patient entering a A&E resus is something special. I don't mean it is entertaining to watch, I mean it's an impressive and shocking array of medical terminology and equipment flying everywhere and before you know it a hundred and one things have been tested and completed in order to help this patient. I stood there trying to listen and learn about what they were saying and watched in awe at all the techniques as they were trying to get her heart rate back to a normal rhythm – none of which was working. Sadly, I think things were getting worse. As I stood there hearing the concerned voices of the nurses and doctors, praying that her heart would just snap back into normal rhythm I felt a tap on my shoulder. It's the little girl's mother.

'Are you OK?' I ask comfortingly.

'Yes thanks, erm… can I go back home? I need to get my other child." She looks at me as if she has just asked to go home from work early.

'I don't need to give you permission whether or not to stay, but I would advise you to stay. Your child is quite poorly and is going to be very scared and needs you here.'

'Oh, OK, well I need to make some phone calls.' She left the resus room with her phone in her hand. I watched as she left and heard the screams and cries from her daughter and just wished she would come and hug her child.

We are just human beings. Our emotions and ability to handle stressful situations differs immensely, so you can never really judge someone for their actions. But at that moment in the heat of it, I did judge. I wanted to shout at this woman to sort out her priorities, as her child could die at any minute and she would never forgive herself if she was out on the phone at the time and not by her side!

If I'm honest now, reflecting back on it, the mother may have not understood the danger her child was in and thought it was OK to leave her side. I found out later that this little girl was rushed to Great Ormond Street Hospital for an emergency open heart surgery.

I will never know if she survived or not.

25

Is It Just A Bit Of Anxiety

At this point I had only ever seen children in SVT (supraventricular tachycardia) for some reason. I had one other case and that was a 16-year-old boy. We picked him up from school as he had been complaining of chest pain and had felt his heart racing. According to school's staff, he looked pale. When we got to him, he did look pale indeed. The school's staff were standing around looking extremely concerned. My first thought was: *Let's just check his heart rate first,* to rule out the possibility that anything serious was going on. I was surprised to feel his heartbeat pounding away at a rate of 240 bpm. We grabbed a chair and got him into the back of the ambulance. A few short minutes later we had rigged him up to all our equipment so now he looked like a cyborg. Then his father arrived on the truck.

'You having another episode, son?'

'Yeah,' he looked sad and fed up.

'So, what's making him feel this way? Is it just a bit of anxiety?' asked the father to us.

'No Sir, definitely not, your son is in something called SVT. His heart rate is at 240 bpm. He should be around 80 give or take. You say another episode, how many times has this happened?'

'Quite a few times now, he just tells us that he feels his heart is racing. We've just been telling him to calm down and breathe through it.'

'OK, well he needs medical treatment for this and probably a treatment plan going forward to stop it from happening. So, we're going to pop him up to the hospital in a few minutes. The father looked at me and then his son.

'Does he need to go? Last time it stopped on its own after a few hours.'

'A few hours! Sir, his heart is a muscle and if it works at this rate for so long it will eventually just give out. It's not meant to work like this. He needs to be in hospital.'

'Oh right, OK, well can I drive up behind you so I have the car.'

'Yeah sure, we will look after him.' Now at this point my crewmate and I decided to try a few tricks we had learned to reverse SVT on adults.

They go like this. Get a 20ml syringe and get the patient to blow as hard as they can for as long as they can. This is called the Valsalva Manoeuvre and, essentially, without going into cardiac output and stroke volumes it causes the heart to arrest the super ventricular tachycardia. However, this didn't help to normalise his heart rate. So, we then went and tried the modified Valsalva, which is doing the same thing with a syringe, but tilting the body back and raising the legs at the same time to create a seesaw effect. You feel like you're grasping at straws when you're rocking a boy back and forth on a stretcher bed –

but it bloody worked!

We watched the screen with anticipation as we flung him back, 240… 240… 240… we were still waiting with his legs in the air and then all of a sudden: 210…. 180… 150… 120… 100…. I felt like we had just performed magic and it was bloody cool!

My crewmate and I gave ourselves a little high-five as we crossed paths trying to hide the fact that we were really bloody chuffed that it had actually worked! And off we popped to hospital with the young boy now feeling a million times better.

It amazes me how the body works – I have so much respect for it that it kind of terrifies me. The body is so complex and wondrous that you would be incredibly naïve to think that you really 100% know what's going on in each cell, each atom and each electrical impulse. So, when I manage to fix someone, all I can call it is *magic.* Other clinicians call it clinical-based evidence and research but, hey, I think magic sounds better.

26

Let's Lighten The Mood Shall We

This book is unfortunately probably going to finish off on some of my worst jobs to date, as they have taught me the most. They have reduced me to tears and made me reflect on my job in a different light. So, before I do that, how about a list of some of the jobs that have made me smile for so many different reasons?

CALL: Numbness in hands and feet

'Every time it gets cold, my hands and feet go numb. It only goes away when I put gloves and warm socks on. I always have to have the heating on, and it's costing me a fortune!' – yes, she called an ambulance out because she was cold!

CALL: Difficulty in swallowing

The gentleman had actually had the problem for some years, so I'm not sure why he called that night. But the wife was a lovely, small Indian lady, and after we had helped her husband

and told him he could stay at home, she decided to bring us a buffet of home-cooked Indian food at three in the morning. I had never tasted onion bhajis quite like it in my life, and it was all washed down with freshly squeezed mango juice and pudding! Just amazing.

CALL: Catastrophic haemorrhaging

Lost finger in kitchen accident? A fall down the stairs? Well, no, the guy smashed a plate and a shard cut a 0.5 cm laceration to his forefinger. Apparently, it wouldn't stop bleeding so he got scared. We walked out soon after walking in. Enough said.

CALL: Elder fallen behind closed doors

We were called to the address of an elderly lady who had become unresponsive and hadn't been seen all day by her care team. Basically, she hadn't answered the door and carers do not have keys. So, we arrived and, of course, got no answer. We needed to make sure she was OK before leaving so this only meant one thing: break the door down. We called the police to aid us. They couldn't break the door down. So, we called the fire department. They broke the door down as well as breaking a window and half of the structural frame around the door. Along with this we had an ambulance, a police car, and a fire engine filling the street which had attracted a crowd of onlookers. To make matters worse, the property was in a block of flats so everyone could see from their windows, so we really did have an audience. We finally got into the property to find that the flat was indeed empty and was clearly not owned by an elderly lady. We confirmed the property address to control and it turns out the care company had sent the wrong address. The elderly lady in question was quite comfortable sitting in her actual home with a cup of tea when police arrived. However, at this address, someone was going to be coming home from work to a smashed-up front door and no kitchen window.

Check your information, people!

CALL: Burning chest

We were called to a 32-year-old woman who had ate curry earlier in the evening and was now suffering with a burning sensation coming from her stomach to her throat. It was described as 'a fire travelling up her windpipe.'

Hmm, could it be heartburn, Miss?

CALL: Unable to cope

We were called to a middle-aged man who was complaining that the state of untidiness he was living in was causing him to have mental health issues. We explained GP referrals and strategies to help this guy. GP's are a great place to start if you feel you are struggling with your mental health. They have an abundance of resources to direct you to the best help.

'What about a cleaner once a week? Do you think that will help you out with your work schedule?'

'Well, can't you guys just do it? I mean that's why I called...'

'...'

That's the sound of my jaw hitting the ground...

CALL: Matern-i-taxi

Definition: When a woman thinks she is in labour and doesn't want to pay for a taxi to the hospital.

CALL: Chest pain

'So, I stood up and stretched and then felt my muscle twitch in my chest and it hurt.'

'Right? Is the pain still there?'

'No, it's gone now, but I think I should go to the hospital.'

'Why did you not jump in a taxi, if you were concerned?'

'Oh, I didn't think of that.'

WHEN NOT TO CALL

My Dad was once in a car accident, it involved him in his car and a lorry. The lorry had tried to move over into the middle lane of a motorway. Unfortunately, this driver didn't see my Dad's car in his blind shoulder and clipped the back left-hand side of the car. This caused Dad's car to slide right into the path of the lorry. The car was immediately a write-off and my Dad was left with a pretty banged up arm. So, there was my Dad in the evening with a self-made sling holding up his possibly broken arm, and good arm holding his tea. 'I'm not going to the hospital. Am I dying? No, so I don't need to be there. I will go to my GP if it doesn't start feeling better soon.' This is how I remember being raised. Go to the hospital if things get really bad, otherwise GO TO YOUR GP! Maybe don't follow my Dad's advice - if you think you have broken your arm, please go to A&E.

27

It Just Seems To Creep Up On You

I'm afraid this is the part where my story gets a little dark. When I say dark, I mean, it involves anxiety, exhaustion, not sleeping, and even nightmares. I didn't get into this job with such naivety that I thought it would always be smooth sailing, that things wouldn't get to me or that I wouldn't feel stress. However, I've never been prone to stress as a person. I have always been able to compartmentalise my work from my home life, and switch off as soon as I get home. At the beginning I was doing this quite nicely. I could finish my day's work and drive home with a smile on my face and be ready for the evening plans. I can't fully recall when the turning point was, when work started coming home with me.

It is there from the moment I wake up to the moment I fall asleep. I replay jobs in my mind before I go to sleep and imagine the worst-case scenario and how I would change things. I replay the scenes of some of my worst patients and relive the fear I had at the time. It is frustrating because I try so hard to push it out of my head, especially at night time. I can feel the cogs turning over and over until I can't fit any more words or thoughts into my head.

It wasn't one big horrendous job that tipped me over the edge from coping quite nicely to being in quite a dark place – it was a run of bad jobs over a few weeks. It started with my worst job to date, and spiralled from there to where I am now, at the time of writing this: quiet, reserved, snappy, and wanting to be on my own. There is the constant feeling of heaviness on my chest. I know it is that job that started my decline, but I'm not ready to take it out of my brain and put it onto paper just yet. This may come as a bit of a shock, seeing as I'm writing this book, but I don't actually like talking too much about things that upset me. Because why would you want to always talk about something that upsets you?! It doesn't make sense to me, but the adult in me knows that it is how to deal with something.

I have spoken to loved ones and relayed my feelings. But I'm a couple of months down the road now and to them it is all forgotten and we have all moved on. At the end of the day: 'it's all part of the job.' It has completely changed how I feel and act when I'm at work. I'm exhausted from lack of sleep and when I do have some time off work, I spend this time dreading going back to work. I know this is not how you're supposed to live your life. Everyone needs a work/life balance, but I'm afraid my scales have tipped over and fallen on the floor and now they are broken.

Today is a Sunday; a cold grey November day, and after the last two weeks of night shifts and even more stress I can feel my emotions boil to the top and finally spill over into my personal life. My partner and I are arguing and sniping at each other, and none of it is his fault. It's mine completely; it makes me even more guilty that I can't seem to keep my emotions in check and leave them in the confines of work!

So today I have decided to take myself away and write these feelings down. Will it make me feel better?

I've no idea, but I've got to try something.

28

It Will Be Ok Sweetie

This is it. This was the job that caused my first mini-breakdown at work. I'm actually finding it hard to know where to start describing it, so I'll just start from the beginning.

I was on a night shift and I was driving the first half of it. Up to this point, me and the crewmate I was working with that evening had been to the most ridiculous jobs, one of which I mentioned earlier. Numb hands and feet when she was feeling cold! We also had a headache. No, not a mind-blistering migraine that feels like someone has hit you round the back of the head with a baseball bat... no, just a normal headache. Also, no, they had not taken any pain relief. Anyway, I digress.

We had come to the halfway point of the shift and it was time to swap over, so now I would attend and my crewmate would drive. I jumped into the attendant's seat and I quite clearly remember saying: 'Watch, I'm about to get all the fucked up, weird jobs.'

My crewmate laughed and agreed, because up to this point

the night had been blissful and easy. Then the job came in – on the screen it read: *10-year-old with brain CA and DIB.* Difficulty in breathing can be so many different things, from chesty coughs, heart conditions, and actually struggling to breathe, all the way to not breathing at all. I had a feeling in my gut that this job was going to be horrendous and I started to panic. I remember I started to sweat all over my body. I flicked quickly through my guidebook to see basic calculations for a 10-year-old as a precaution in case I needed them, but also, I believe it was to keep me busy while driving to this job – so I didn't freak out too much in my mind. I was praying that it really wasn't as bad as it sounded. We arrived on the scene and saw the house with the lights on. We jumped out and grabbed our stuff from the truck and started to head to the door. The door was opened by an elderly lady. Her Nan maybe?

'Hi, are we at the right address?'

'Yes, come in, it's that door on the left.' She said this with no real hesitation in her voice. It almost had an air of calm, as if she was inviting me round for tea. My nerves wavered a fraction, thinking that maybe my prayers had been answered and the little girl was not as bad as I had imagined. I walked into the room, where she is lying on the sofa wrapped in a blanket, with Mum sitting by her feet and Dad standing by her side. They were both staring at me. I took one look at the little girl and knew straight away that this was not going to be OK. She was seriously ill and wasn't just having difficulty with her breathing – she was barely breathing at all. But God, she was trying with all her might. Her eyes were fixed on mine the whole time, and with every effort of her body as she tried to take a breath, I could see her eyes becoming more bloodshot.

I grabbed the device that measures oxygen levels and chucked it on her finger while asking for high flow oxygen to be set up immediately. Grabbing my stethoscope as quickly as I could I had a listen to her chest and heard nothing: no intake of breath and none out. Her chest was moving, but the air wasn't moving. The oxygen was on and I finally looked up at her parents to say we were going.

'Are you Dad?'

'Me? Yes.'

'OK Dad, grab her, we need to go now.' Mum replied by explaining that the girl had cancer and had been having a coughing fit, then vomited.

'Is she nil by mouth?' This means you cannot swallow food, and have your food through a peg feed. This is essentially a tube that is inserted directly into your stomach and liquid full of nutrients and the vitamins that you need are pumped into your stomach just like you getting a meal.

'Yes,' Mum replied. Dad has still not picked up his daughter. By this point I have grabbed her myself, picked her up in my arms and told her everything was going to be OK. She had aspirated on her own vomit. In simpler terms, she was choking on her vomit and it had now gone into her lungs, preventing the air from entering and exchanging properly, which is what breathing essentially is.

She couldn't breathe. It was clear in my mind that she was dying but how long did we have? The Dad looked at me in confusion as to why I was struggling to hold this 10-year-old girl in my arms and hold the oxygen canister while my crewmate carried, or I should say, ran the bags out to the truck.

'Do you want me to carry her?'

'Yes, take her and let's go out to the truck now. Mum, are you coming?'

'Yes yes, I'll grab a bag.'

'OK, PLEASE BE QUICK!' I yelled as we left the house; it was my calmest but most serious yell yet. The kind of yell that means: *Don't panic but get a bloody move on.* My hands were shaking like a leaf while we connected this girl to the machines in the truck. Were we going to get a better reading or worse? I just didn't know at this point; her oxygen levels were unreadable and her heart rate high.

I also stuck on something called a capnography, which counts the number of breaths you do in one minute and displays it on the screen. It also showed me every time my patient took a breath. I looked at the rise and fall of her chest, which was shaky and erratic. I looked at the monitor and she was breathing at a rate of 22 breaths per minute. However, she was starting to develop cyanosis on her face and limbs. I shouted through the truck for my crewmate to start driving and put a blue call in to the nearest hospital, alerting them that this patient has severe DIB, and handing over what little observations I had.

When handing over a blue call to a hospital they want to know as much information as possible, which of course makes sense. They want to know temperatures, sugar levels, blood pressure, pupil size, heart rate, resp rate, GCS, all these things… but for this little girl we simply didn't have time. It was grab and go. There was nothing more I could do for her and she needed the hospital.

We started to head off and it was the first time I noticed that her mother was sitting in the chair beside me. We could have left without her, honestly, I had no awareness of anything around me apart from this patient and the machine she was attached to. I was standing by her head and looked down to see her eyes still locked onto mine: they were deep red now. I could see the veins in her eyes like little red lightning bolts and within them this sheer look of panic.

The machine beeped. I swung my head round to see the orange line that showed me her respiratory effort had flattened out. The counter now read four breaths a minute. I threw off the fluffy blanket that the little girl was wrapped in, as Mum hadn't wanted her to get cold, and I stared at her chest. It can only have been a couple of seconds, but it felt like ages. I checked the monitor, then I checked her. Was she breathing?

I placed a hand on the centre of her chest to feel the rise and fall and there was none. Fuck. Diving over the other side of the truck I grabbed a BVM (bag valve mask) and started manually ventilating her, or should I say, assisting in her breathing. I placed the mask over her face and started quickly stroking the side of her cheek to let her know it was going to be OK. I press down on the bag and I see her chest start to rise. In all the panic I keep running through this question in my head: *Is this the right thing to do?*

'WHAT'S GOING ON?' shouted my crewmate, who was still driving through the busy London traffic.

'Her resps dropped so I'm bagging.'

'Jesus, you OK, you need me to pull over?'

'No, no keep going...' A million things were running through my head: *Should I be doing something else? Have I missed anything? God, am I killing this little girl? Should I be putting on a neb? But if she can't breathe then a neb won't help?* All of this was going on while I was staring at her, then at the monitor, then back at her eyes.

'It's OK, I'm sorry, I'm trying to help you breathe sweetie. We will be at the hospital soon and they will make you better. They have all the lovely, nice doctors and nurses there who will make you better.' I said this quietly, and in my calmest, sweetest voice, kept speaking to the little girl while she stared up at me. As my flushed, sweaty face hung over hers, I felt the truck pull up at the hospital. We were here. Thank God. *Go go go!*

We rushed her into resus, where the team was waiting in the paediatric bay for us. A nurse caught sight of us walking in and saw me bagging the little girl, who was floppy. She ran over to lend a hand, which we accepted with much appreciation. She was quickly transferred onto the other bed. There was no need for a detailed handover for this patient. I transferred the BVM to one of the nurses and stated 'She has brain CA, nil by mouth, aspirated on vomit. Lost respiratory effort en route.'

At that I stepped back. I could do no more. I stood on the side-lines and watched as the nurses and doctors swarmed around her and I prayed that I had made the right decisions. The mother was standing not too far from me, I felt particularly guilty when the nurse came up to me (and not the mother), placed a hand on my shoulder and said: 'Are you OK?' This wasn't the generic 'Are you OK?' It wasn't like the way you would say it as when meeting up with someone for coffee or over the phone. This was more like: 'You look like are about to crumble and I'm worried about you.'

I responded by simply looking at her and nodding. Half a smile and then I knew it. I had to walk out. I was about to lose it and, dammit, I wasn't going to lose it in front of the staff, the mother and, most of all, the patient. I quickly walked outside back to where the ambulances were and let the tears come. Hard, heavy and relentless.

I have never to this day experienced fear like that in my life. To stand completely in charge of another person's life while it teetered between life and death. Especially someone so young.

It broke me in ways I didn't know it could. I couldn't talk, I couldn't think. I had shut down. All the adrenaline had left my body and I had no more tears left to cry. (At that point anyway.) As a result, I had to take some time off the road as I would have been a danger to any other patient if I were in charge of their care. It was only a couple of hours but it was enough to begin functioning again.

The entire job, from arriving on scene to arriving at hospital, had taken 17 minutes.

I called my boyfriend in the early hours of that morning and cried down the phone. I didn't need to speak. I just needed to cry to someone who knew me and loved me instead of crying to myself sitting up against a brick wall.

All I wanted to do was to go home to him and hold him in my arms. Crawl into my bed and stay there, where it was safe – and not be sitting on the streets of London by myself. I tried to ring my Mum, who is my security blanket, but she was fast asleep and didn't pick up the phone.

I remember sitting there and thinking to myself: *Why the hell did I choose this job, this responsibility, this path for my life when there were so many other choices I could have made?* Most of all, *Could I keep doing this until I retire? Could my mind hack it or will it just consume me and make me this numb, walking organism?*

I drove home that morning reliving the scene I had experienced, asking myself: *Did I do that right, should I have done that first?* Her eyes were the last thing I remembered when I fell asleep that morning. Her eyes looking back at me the whole time. I had to go back the following night and do it all again. I still don't quite know how I did that. But I was there and back on the truck within 12 hours. This was followed by two months of relentless blue calls, sick kids and serious jobs.

Which all finished with a week of seven blue calls that led to a weekend of anxiety attacks and mild to acute depression.

Here's a taste of my week of blue calls:

29

I Can't Stand Up

This elderly gentleman lived on the third floor with no lift. Let's start off there, shall we? Might I also add that this elderly gentleman weighed 21 stone. First problem.

Second problem was he was also in SVT (supraventricular tachycardia) with a heart rate of 230 bpm. He was breathing at a rate of 38 bpm. He was sweating profusely and correctly informed us he couldn't stand, as he felt like he was going to pass out – and I'm not surprised. He needed to be carried out, but we couldn't do it alone. We needed help. We called for an extra member of staff to assist us down the stairs. But while we were waiting for assistance to arrive, it all started going horribly wrong.

We already had the ECG dots in place on this man's chest so we could see his heart rhythm on the screen of our monitor. It was showing a narrow complex SVT. *OK, I can deal with this,* I thought. We got a blood pressure reading and it was on the low side of normal. Which is probably why he would have felt dizzy when standing. When he was sitting it was manageable, so just to err on the safe side of caution I decided to get a line in (meaning to place a cannula into his arm) just in case we needed fluids. My crewmate had to run back down the three flights of stairs as we had no 20ml syringes in our med packs to try the Valsalva technique.

So off he ran and while I was setting up my cannula roll ready to place the needle in his arm another BP showed up on the screen: it was now 69/40. Crap. This had dropped dramatically, so I had to get the line in as quickly as possible and start running fluids. To my complete surprise, I managed to get an 18g cannula in first time and quickly prepped the fluids. My crewmate came back into the flat, breathless and sweaty, at which moment I shoved the fluids into his face to cross-check the drug and dates. He agreed they were good to go and I started to run the fluids.

Another BP showed up onto the screen: it was now 61/39. I squeezed the bag to make the fluid enter his bloodstream as quickly as possible, but then something caught my eye. His narrow complex SVT (his heart rhythm) had now changed. It now looked like a rhythm called VT. If you don't know what this looks like, I would advise you to do a quick Google search and see how bizarre it is. Another key point to this VT rhythm is that people in VT are often DEAD. It is one of the rhythms we shock in cardiac arrest, so you can imagine I quickly looked at my patient, then back at the monitor, and back at my patient.

'Erm, Steve are you seeing this?' I gestured to the monitor and we quickly printed a rhythm strip so we could prove our eyes weren't deceiving us.

'Yes, that is definitely VT.' I was still squeezing the fluid bag and thankfully his blood pressure was on the rise. I looked again at the monitor and now he was back in SVT. He was still sweating profusely and becoming tired, not surprisingly as the poor man was breathing at the rate of 40bpm. The extra help arrived and we got him down to the truck. We connected him to the machines in the truck and, believe it or not, his heart rate was now stabilised. His rhythm complexes were back to a normal range too.

'Are you feeling better now, Sir?'

'Yes, loads, thank you.' I felt bad accepting his thanks as we didn't really do much, but his symptoms seemed to have self-resolved and I was ecstatic.

We blued him into the nearest hospital, purely because of the fact that his heart rhythm had been doing some weird and wonderful things while we were on the scene. Thankfully the doctor agreed with our decision to bring him straight into resus and not normal ED – and you know you've brought something strange into the resus doctors when they huddle around an ECG and pull strange faces.

30

Mummy Can't Breathe

L ater that day we got a job sent to us of a 'woman struggling to breathe.' In the notes it stated there were kids on the scene.

We arrived at this job and I could tell which home we were attending by the young boy, around eight years old, waving at us from the door. We jumped out of the truck and grabbed our kit as usual. Walking into the property, I immediately saw a middle-aged woman lying on her side along the stairs gasping for breath.

The boy told me that she had asthma. Crying in the background was a three-year-old girl and, quite oblivious to the mayhem, was a barely two-year-old little boy playing with his toys in the living room. I realise now that the son had put the call to 999 through as his mother could barely breathe, let alone speak.

We quickly made our way over to her and applied a nebuliser filled with salbutamol and ipratropium bromide after listening to the horrendous wheeze inside her lungs. The bases of her lungs were quiet from so much inflammation and constriction. Her oxygen levels were in the 60s. She was having such a bad asthma attack that we had to consider it to be life-threatening asthma. She was clammy, pale, unable to speak in between breaths and using every muscle she could to breathe. We quickly decided this was the route we were going down, so I drew up some IM (intramuscular) adrenaline. For life-threatening asthma, adrenaline relieves the bronchospasm that is happening in your lungs.

Then we moved onto hydrocortisone IV (intravenous), which suppresses the inflammation and immune response. Her oxygen levels were improving but were still at a dangerous level, so it was time to pack up and get out to the truck as quickly as possible. All we could do at that point was to continue with the nebuliser and hope the drugs started taking effect. We left with the patient in the carry chair, a two-year-old in one arm, bags in another. The other two children were holding hands and crying to get to Mummy. We made our way out to the truck to begin heading off to hospital. We only have three seats in the back of an ambulance, of which one is equipped with a baby seat. So, with time not on our side, we had to secure three screaming children in their selected seats, and secure Mum who was still struggling away. Then there was me, with no seat left. I had to manage the patient, monitor her levels and continue treatment, all while playing the surfing game in a moving vehicle. During transport the patient had improved enough to hand me her phone with a contact on the screen; she was pointing at the number and then to her children. I took this to mean: 'Please call this woman to get the kids.' I asked her if this is what she meant and I was right, so now I was arranging child pickups as well as everything else. The patient was right, however. The children were going to need someone with them when we arrived at the hospital as Mum was going to be rather busy.

The friend reacted just as my Mum would have, and that was by flapping and screaming at her husband to get the keys. I tried to calm her as much as I could but I guess the kids screaming in the background scared her enough to not really listen to what I was saying – which I completely understand.

The journey to hospital was around 8-10 minutes and as we are pulling into the entrance to the hospital, I noticed my patient taking long deep breaths. The kind you take when you have finally completely a relentless task. 'Are you OK?' I shouted at her over the children.

She started to cry and, as tears rolled down her face she smiled and nodded her head: 'Yes, better.' She smiled again and reached out a hand to her eldest boy to say: 'I'm okay now.' The little boy began to cry while holding his Mum's hand. Then it dawned on me. I had been so busy treating the patient and doing my job that I hadn't taken into account the fact that this woman would have been terrified for her life. She would have thought she was dying and if it hadn't been for her little boy calling the ambulance then maybe she would have done. She was crying with joy and relief. Her son had saved her life.

We handed the patient over into resus and the doctor looked over the treatment plan we had given, what the original vital signs had been and where they now sat. The doctor went over to the patient, who was smiling but still clearly struggling and he said: 'Well I think it's safe to say that these guys just saved your life.'

That single sentence felt like a slap in the face, but in a good way. I remember my face getting hot and wishing he hadn't

151

said it. I'm not too sure why, because that's got to be the single most amazing thing someone can say about you – but at the time, with the patient smiling and thanking me and reaching out for my hand to hold, I just wanted to shrivel up and hide so no one could look at me. I smiled back, squeezed her hand and made my way out to the truck to finish my paperwork. I just needed five minutes of quiet to digest what had just happened.

NOT EVERYONE HAS PEOPLE AROUND THEM

A couple of days later we got called to an elderly lady who had become unresponsive in a care home. A car was already on the scene but we arrived shortly after it. I took one look at the monitor that the medic had already attached to the patient and noticed that her blood pressure was extremely low and her heart rate was at a steady rate of 24bpm. Not good. The carer came up to me and showed me a DNR form that was in this lady's care folder. Skipping ahead a little bit, we had got her onto the truck and had already begun treatment for her symptoms. While en route to the hospital, I was in the back with the patient on my own and watching to see if the medication was taking effect.

It dawned on me at this point, that if this lady was going to die, I would just have to stand there and watch it happen. She was alone, with no family by her side. She had no idea what was happening to her. It was just me and her. I would have to watch as her heart stopped beating and wait until her heart completely stopped... then I could call time of death.

This is not how any person should leave this world and I prayed that the medication would start to work. I watched as her heart rate slowly increased, and her blood pressure was doing the same. The patient came round enough on the journey to hospital that I could actually have a conversation with her. I smiled at her as she asked if her family would be there at the hospital.

'Yes, the carers were calling your son when we left your home.' I held her hand the whole way. I knew she might not have long left but at least she would be surrounded by her family when the time came, and not in the back of my ambulance.

31

All In A Days Work

My week finished off with a four-month-old with meningitis; a 10-year-old with life-threatening asthma; a two-year-old anaphylaxis, a 50-year-old male wanting to commit suicide while holding a knife to his throat; and a 45-year-old gentleman with severe sepsis who was in peri-arrest. I was completely drained by the end of it, yet I had performed some of my best work and I was getting braver and more confident every day.

Despite all this I had reached a point where I could go on no further. I had just finished a job when I broke down in tears and could not carry on my shift. I was reported for welfare and a meeting was arranged with my managers. After balling my eyes out for nearly two hours, I was signed off work for two months. I applied for counselling and was quickly diagnosed with PTSD and depression. After a long battle with myself and learning every self-help technique I could muster I started to feel better. I had the support of my family and friends and LAS to get me through it which I am so grateful for! I was scared to go back to work due to the fears of my past emotions creeping back into my life. Until the coronavirus pandemic hit the UK. Then I knew I had to go back and begin my job again.

In 2020 I am now in my second year as a qualified paramedic working out of London, and blimey has time flown! I look back to where I was during my days as a student and I do feel so proud how far I have come. I am incredibly proud of the work I do, and it isn't just for the fast, adrenaline-filled jobs: it's for the care referrals I do on a day-to-day basis, and the help I can arrange for an elderly patient to live a more comfortable life. It is about safeguarding and raising awareness for children if something is not right at home.

I have to remind myself of these things when it seems all too dark. This job is surrounded by darkness and light and I believe you need to appreciate and respect both aspects. Accept the darkness – but overcome it with the light. The ladies and gentlemen employed in healthcare work relentlessly every day just to make a difference in someone's life. And it is not for the money or the glory. I believe it is because there is no greater honour in this life than to help others when they really need it.

I still on a daily basis have the love and support of my family and friends and I am forever grateful for that! My partner, Chris and I are talking about bringing another little Nash into the world and I can not wait for our next adventure together. My parents are forever my role models and my agony aunts and I wouldn't change a thing about them. They are simply perfect.

My final parting word to you all is this: The world could be a kinder place, but this is the world we live in. So, embrace it, thrive in it, and most of all – enjoy the ride. Just don't forget to hold on through the bumps.

About the Author

I am a paramedic working in London. This consist of early mornings, late nights and enough Redbull to sink a battleship but I love it and couldn't see myself doing any other job. I always wanted to write a book but never felt I had anything to say. My partner showed me I had plenty to say I just needed a push in the right direction.

Printed in Great Britain
by Amazon